Drug-Drug Interactions in the Metabolic Syndrome

DRUG-DRUG INTERACTIONS IN THE METABOLIC SYNDROME

GIANLUCA IACOBELLIS

Nova Science Publishers, Inc.
New York

For permission to use material from this book please contact us:
Telephone 631-231-7269; Fax 631-231-8175
Web Site: http://www.novapublishers.com

Library of Congress Cataloging-in-Publication Data
Iacobellis, Gianluca.
Drug-drug interactions in the metabolic syndrome / Gianluca Iacobellis.
p. ; cm.
Includes bibliographical references and index.
ISBN 1-59454-952-4
. Metabolic syndrome--Chemotherapy--Complications. 2. Drug interactions.
[DNLM: 1. Metabolic Syndrome X--drug therapy. 2. Anti-Obesity Agents--pharmacokinetics. 3. Antilipemic Agents--pharmacokinetics. 4. Drug Interactions. 5. Hypoglycemic Agents--pharmacokinetics. WK 820 I11d 2006] I. Title.
RC662.4.I23 2006
616.3'9061--dc22 2006000069

Published by Nova Science Publishers, Inc. ✦New York

CONTENTS

AUTHOR'S BIOGRAPHY

Gianluca Iacobellis MD, PhD, obtained his medical degree, specialty and post doctoral degree in Endocrinology and Metabolic Disorders at La Sapienza University, Rome, Italy. He is currently Clinical Research Fellow in the Department of Medicine, Cardiovascular Obesity Research and Management, McMaster University, Hamilton General Hospital, ON, Canada. Until the beginning of 2005, he was Post Doctoral Clinical Research Fellow at the Center for Human Nutrition University of Texas Southwestern Medical Center at Dallas. Dr Iacobellis has authored several papers and lectured worldwide on the cardiovascular aspects of obesity and metabolic syndrome. He is peer-reviewer of cardiology and endocrinology journals.

INTRODUCTION AND AIM

THE METABOLIC SYNDROME

Metabolic syndrome is a cluster of multiple cardiovascular risk factors. In fact, Metabolic Syndrome is defined by the presence of the following alterations: 1) obesity, (mainly visceral adiposity), 2) hypertension, 3) impaired glucose tolerance (impaired fasting glucose, glucose intolerance or diabetes) and 4) dyslipidaemia (tables 1 and 2). Which among insulin resistance, central obesity and lipid abnormalities is the key factor of metabolic syndrome is still controversial [1-3]. Probably, the concomitant presence of each different variable plays the crucial role in developing the metabolic syndrome. Since lowered cut-off points of waist circumference, used as marker of abdominal adiposity, and fasting glucose have been recently proposed [3] it is intuitive that the prevalence of Metabolic Syndrome will increase (tables 1 and 2). When lifestyle changes and dietetic recommendations fail to improve the poor metabolic profile of the patient affected by metabolic syndrome a pharmacological treatment is necessary. However, since the patient with metabolic syndrome presents multiple metabolic and cardiovascular alterations, a multiple drug therapy is often performed. Therefore, drug-drug interaction could occur when two or more drugs are concomitantly administrated. Some of these drug-drug interactions are well known whereas others could be underestimated or unknown.

This book seeks to report updated data from the literature on the potential drug-drug interactions occurring between drugs used to treat each individual disease of metabolic syndrome. The manual is focused on the metabolic syndrome drugs. Possible drug-drug interactions and their potential mechanisms are summarized and discussed. Chemical characteristics and mechanisms of action of each drug are also briefly described. Some new anti-obesity, anti-diabetes, lipid lowering and anti-hypertensive drugs are also reported and briefly discussed. This book can be a practical manual for the specialist, the practioner and also the clinical researcher.

Table 1. Metabolic syndrome components according to ATPIII definition

• Abdominal obesity (elevated waist circumference) *Men > 102 cm; Women > 88 cm*
• Raised triglycerides (> 150 mg/dL)
• Reduced HDL cholesterol *Men < 40 mg/dL; Women < 50 mg/dL*
• Raised blood pressure (> 130/ or > 85)
• Elevated plasma glucose (> 110 mg dl)

Table 2. Metabolic syndrome components according to IDF definition

• Central obesity *Men > 94 cm; Women > 80 cm* *Plus any two of the following four factors:*
• Raised triglycerides (> 150 mg/dL)
• Reduced HDL cholesterol *Men < 40 mg/dL; Women < 50 mg/dL*
• Raised blood pressure (> 130/ or > 85)
• Elevated plasma glucose (> 100 mg dl)

References

[1] Grundy SM et al. Definition of metabolic syndrome: Report of the National Heart, Lung, and Blood Institute/American Heart Association conference on scientific issues related to definition. *Circulation.* 2004 Jan 27;109(3):433-8.

[2] Grundy SM et al. Implications of recent clinical trials for the National Cholesterol Education Program Adult Treatment Panel III Guidelines. *J Am Coll Cardiol.* 2004 Aug 4;44(3):720-32.

[3] Hanley AJ, Wagenknecht LE, D'Agostino RB Jr, Zinman B, Haffner SM. Identification of subjects with insulin resistance and beta-cell dysfunction using alternative definitions of the metabolic syndrome. *Diabetes.* 2003 Nov;52(11):2740-7.

Chapter 1

DRUG-DRUG INTERACTIONS: BASIC PRINCIPLES OF PHARMACOLOGY

DEFINITION OF DRUG-DRUG INTERACTION

A drug-drug interaction generally occurs when either the pharmacokinetics or pharmacodynamics of one drug is altered by another [1-2].

PHARMACODYNAMIC INTERACTIONS

Pharmacodynamic drug-drug interactions result when one drug alters the sensitivity or responsiveness of tissues to another drug. The drugs may have opposing (antagonistic) or additive pharmacologic effects. Antagonistic effects between two drugs may not be easy to detect. Older patients are especially susceptible, with consequent risk of falls and injuries, although many persons take these combinations without serious problems.

PHARMACOKINETIC INTERACTIONS

Pharmacokinetic interactions may be complicated and difficult to predict. They are mainly due to alteration of drug absorption, distribution, metabolism, or excretion, thereby changing the amount and persistence of available drug at receptor sites. Magnitude and duration, not type, of effect are changed. Pharmacokinetic interactions are often predicted based on knowledge of the individual drugs or detected by monitoring the patient for clinical signs and for changes in serum concentrations of drugs. Pharmacokinetics terms used in this volume are summarized in Table 1.

Drug Interactions Involving Altered Absorption

When the absorption rate of a drug is altered, clinically significant drug interactions are more likely to occur, especially when the drug has a short half-life or it requires a rapid peak plasma drug level to achieve a therapeutic effect. Drug interactions involving a drug's gastrointestinal absorption generally result in a decrease rather than an increase in drug absorption. The mechanisms of action for these interactions include: 1) altered gastrointestinal pH-values; 2) the formation of insoluble complexes or chelated compounds; 3) drugs being bound to bile acid sequestrant drugs; 4) altered gastrointestinal function (acceleration or slowing of gastric emptying, change in vascularity or permeability of gastrointestinal mucosa, or mucosal damage of the gut wall); and 5) altered intestinal blood flow. Of these possible mechanisms of action, most clinically significant drug interactions result from the formation of insoluble complexes, or chelates, and when drugs are bound to resins that bind bile acids. Although it is certainly possible, few clinically significant drug interactions occur as a result of changes in intestinal blood flow or from changes in gastric motility. However, there are some striking drug interactions with drugs that alter gastrointestinal tract pH, i.e., antacids that lead to a significant decrease in drug bioavailability.

Table 1. Pharmacokinetic Parameters

Primary	Secondary	Steady-state
AUC_{0-24} (ng*h/ml) Area under the concentration-time curve collected over 24 hours	t_{max} (h) Maximum plasma concentration	C_{min} (ng/ml) Concentration at time zero of the last day of treatment.
C_{max} (ng/ml) maximum plasma concentration	$t_{1/2}$ (h) terminal half-life	C_{av} (ng/ml) average concentration during a dosing interval, estimated by AUC_{0-24} divided by 24 hours.

Drug Interactions Involving Altered Drug Distribution

Drugs most likely to be involved in clinically significant interactions include those that: 1) are highly protein bound (~90% or greater), 2) are bound in tissues, 3) have a small volume of distribution (Vd), 4) have a low hepatic extraction ratio, 5) have a narrow therapeutic to toxic ratio, 6) have a rapid onset of action, or 7) are administered intravenously.

Drug Interactions Involving Altered Metabolism

Drugs may go through two different metabolic processes, Phase I and Phase II metabolism. In Phase I metabolism, hepatic microsomal enzymes contained in the endothelium of liver cells first oxidize, demethylate, hydrolyze, etc., drugs to render them more water soluble. In Phase II, large water-soluble substances (e.g., glucuronic acid, sulfate) are attached to the drug to form inactive or significantly less active, water-soluble metabolites. Compounds may circulate through one or both phases multiple times until the water-soluble characteristic is present. More clinically significant drug interactions are caused by Phase I hepatic microsomal enzymes rather than by Phase II metabolism. Most drug metabolism takes place in the liver, but other organs, such as the kidneys, lungs and intestinal tract are also involved. Drugs identified as high-extraction drugs are almost entirely metabolized during the first pass through the liver. In general, high-extraction ratio drugs are less affected by interactions than low-extraction drugs. These drugs usually have a short half-life, and their metabolites are usually inactive. However, the lower the therapeutic index of a drug, the more serious the potential consequences of drug interactions affecting metabolism. In some instances, a drug interaction may result from the sequence in which drugs are administered.

Drug Interactions Involving Altered Elimination

Drug interactions that occur at the level of excretion may involve one or more of the following: 1) glomerular filtration, 2) active secretion or passive reabsorption in the renal tubular system, or 3) competition of drugs for the same active transport system. Drugs with the ability to increase or decrease glomerular filtration by altering the renal blood flow may influence the rate of excretion of other drugs or their active or inactive metabolites. For drugs with narrow therapeutic ratios, increasing their renal clearance reduces their plasma steady-state concentrations, whereas interference with the renal excretion mechanisms will increase their circulating level and may result in toxic drug levels. Drug interactions can occur when changes in urinary pH alter the excretion of weakly acidic or weakly basic drugs by affecting their extent of ionization. This consequently affects their reabsorption from the lumen of renal tubules.

Main References

[1] Gibaldi, M. *Pharmacokinetic variability–drug interactions. Biopharmaceutics and clinical pharmacokinetics* (4th ed.), Lea and Febiger, 1991 Philadelphia.

[2] Greenblatt DJ, von Moltke LL. Drug-drug interactions: clinical perspective. In: Rodrigues AD, ed. *Drug-Drug Interactions*. New York: Marcel Dekker; 2002: 565-584.

CYTOCHROME P450

Cytochrome P450 is involved in the metabolism of many drugs used in the metabolic syndrome. Potential drug interactions could be observed between drugs for which CYP450 and Cytochrome P450 Isoenzymes are involved in metabolism (table 2).

Cytochrome P450 catalyzes the oxidation of a wide range of substances from alkanes to alkenes, aromatic rings, thioethers or amines. During the reaction cycle triplet dioxygen is converted to iron-bound activated singlet dioxygen which actually does the oxidation after O-O bond breaking (figure 1)

Table 2. Human Cytochrome P450 Isoenzymes Known to Oxidize Drugs Used in the Metabolic Syndrome

CYP1A2
CYP2C9
CYP2C19
CYP2D6
CYP2E1
CYP3A4
Acetaminophen
Diclofenac
Omeprazole
Flecainide
Acetaminophen
Amiodarone
Fluvastatin
Ibuprofen
Imipramine
Etanol
Atorvastatin
Tolbutamide
Metoprolol
Diltiazem
Warfarin
Mibefradil
Lacidipine
Propafenone
Lovastatin
Propranolol
Mibefradil
Nifedipine
Quinidine
Sildenafil
Simvastatin
Verapamil
Warfarin

Modified from Walsky RL, et al.Examination of 209 drugs for inhibition of cytochrome P450 2C8. J Clin Pharmacol. 2005 Jan;45(1):68-78.

ORGANIC ANION TRANSPORTERS

One of the liver functions is the clearance of a large variety of metabolic products, drugs, and other xenobiotics by transporting them across the sinusoidal membrane into the hepatocyte. Several classes of transport systems have been described that mediate these processes including the Na+/taurocholate cotransporter polypeptide, in rat and human liver, and a family of organic anion transporting polypeptides (OATPs)1 that are principally expressed in liver, kidney, and brain [1]. In contrast to the rat, only one transporter of this family, OATP, has been identified in humans [2]. It is expressed most abundantly throughout the brain and in much lower amounts in liver, kidney, and lung. A liver-specific member of the organic anion transport protein family in humans that mediates the transport of bile acid, the adrenal androgen DHEAS, and HMG-CoA reductase inhibitors, have been identified [2]. In humans, the organic anion transporter OATP2 (also known as OATP-C) is expressed in the liver and makes a substantial contribution to the hepatic uptake of statins, including pravastatin and rosuvastatin [3].

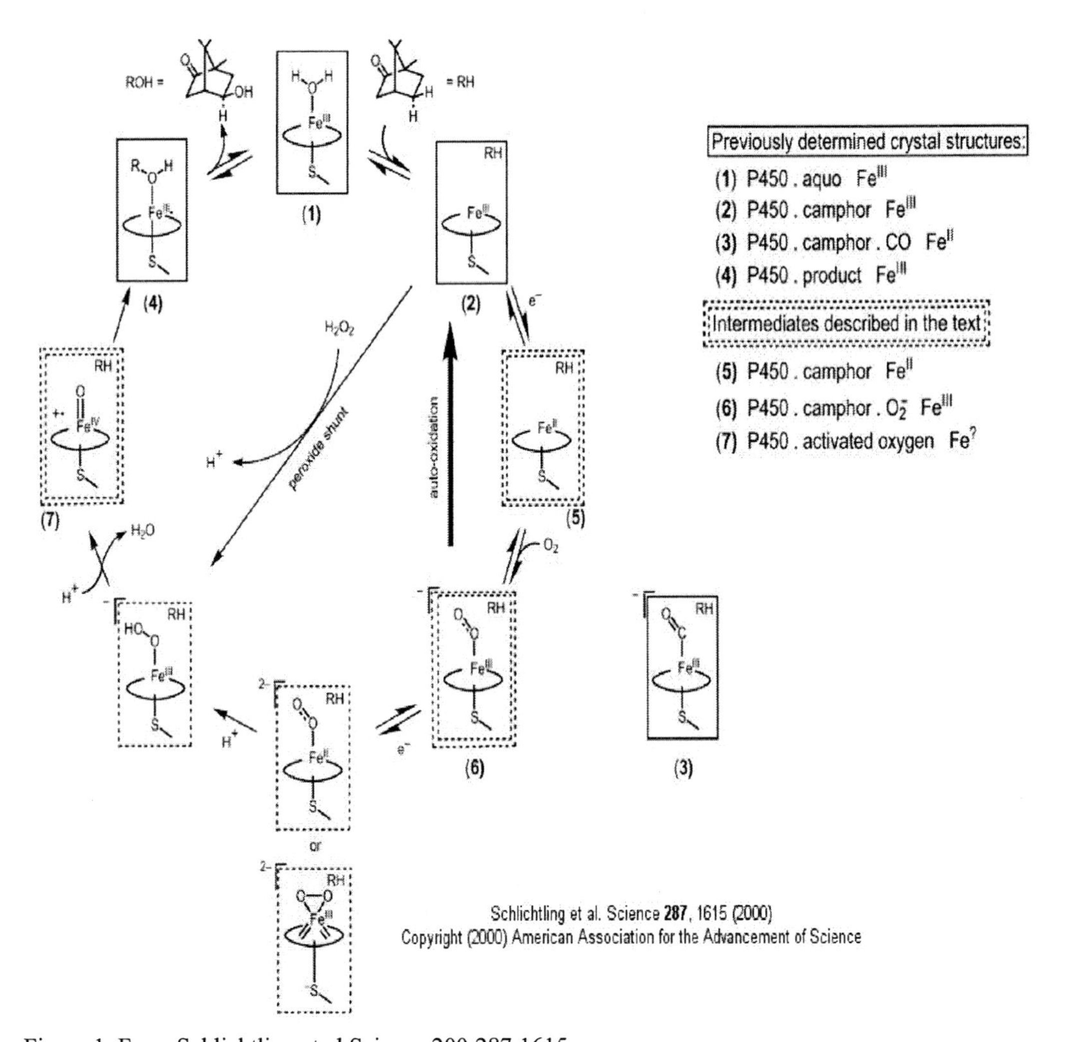

Figure 1. From Schlichtling et al Science 200;287:1615

References

[1] Hagenbuch, B., Stieger, B., Foguet, M., Lubbert, H., and Meier, P. *J. Proc. Natl. Acad. Sci. U. S. A.* 1991; 88, 10629-10633.

[2] Kullak-Ublick, G. A., Hagenbuch, B., Stieger, B., Schteingart, C. D., Hofmann, A. F., Wolkoff, A. W., Meier, P. J. *Gastroenterology* 1995; 109, 1274-1282.

[3] B. Hsiang, Y. Zhu, Z. Wang, Y. Wu, V. Sasseville, W.P. Yang et al., A novel human hepatic organic anion transporting polypeptide (OATP2). *J Biol Chem* 1999,274; 37161–37168.

Chapter 2

ANTI-OBESITY DRUGS

ORLISTAT

Brief Compound Description

Orlistat is (S)-2-formylamino-4-methyl-pentanoic *acid* (S)-1-[[2S, 3S)-3-hexyl-4-oxo-2-oxetanyl] methyl]-dodecyl ester. Its empirical *formula* is $C_{29}H_{53}NO_5$, and its molecular *weight* is 495.7. It is a single diastereomeric *molecule* that contains four chiral centers, with a *negative optical rotation* in *ethanol* at 529 nm. The structural formula is the following:

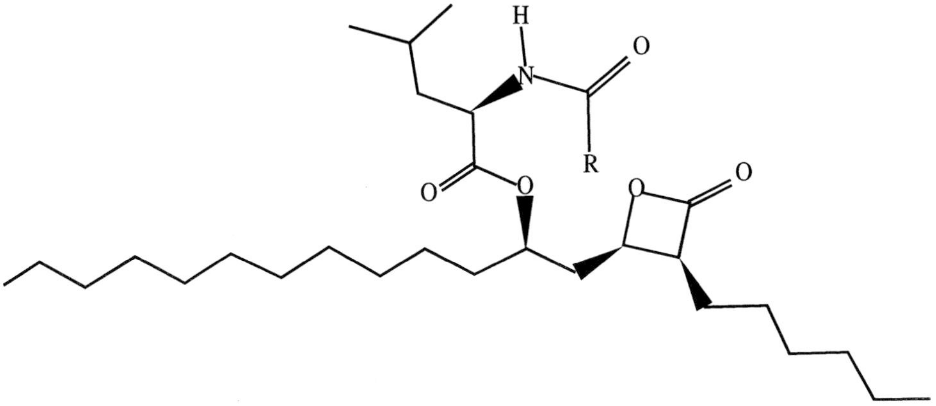

Mechanism of Action

Orlistat is a reversible lipases inhibitor for obesity management that acts by inhibiting the absorption of dietary fats. It acts in the lumen of the stomach and small intestine by forming a covalent bond with the active serine site of gastric and pancreatic lipases. The inactivated enzymes are unavailable to hydrolyze dietary fat in the form of triglycerides into absorbable free fatty acids and monoglycerides. Orlistat inhibits activity of pancreatic and gastric lipases, blocks gastrointestinal uptake of approximately 30% of ingested fat at the dose of 360 mg/daily (120 mg three times a day) [1-4].

Drug Interactions

Due to its mechanism of action, there is the potential of Orlistat to affect the absorption of other drugs, expecially fat soluble drugs. Although several interactions studies have been performed, most of them failed to find drug interactions with orlistat. Main of the possible drug-drug interactions between Orlistat and other components used in patients with metabolic syndrome are summarized in Table 1. Some of these potential interactions are discussed in detail below.

Table 1. Potential drug-drug interactions with Orlistat in metabolic syndrome

YES	mechanism	NO
Amiodarone	↓ Reduced absorption of amiodarone	Atorvastatin, Pravastatin, Simvastatin
Cyclosporine		Losartan Nifedipine
		Digoxin
		Metformin Sibutramine Fluoxetine Glyburide
		Oral contraceptives
		Warfarin

Amitriptylin, atorvastatin, losartan, metformin, phentermine, sibutramine, nifedipine, warfarin, digoxin, glyburide, oral contraceptives, fluoxetine, pravastatin, simvastatin, cerivstatin, and their metabolites were statistically equivalent, therefore unaffected, in presence and absence of orlistat [5-14]. Short-term treatment with orlistat had no significant influence on ethanol pharmacokinetics [12].

Orlistat and Amiodarone

The absorption of amiodarone, highly lipophilic drug, (and active metabolite) was significantly reduced by approximately one-quarter using parameters of Cmax and AUC when orlistat was co-administred. These results indicate that orlistat can affect serum amiodarone concentrations when the two drugs are taken concomitantly [13].

Orlistat and Vitamin E

Orlistat significantly reduced the absorption of vitamin E (approximately 43% according to maximum concentration and approximately 60% according to area under the concentration-time curve), but not that of vitamin A, at the dose levels studied. The results of this study will aid in the implementation of a vitamin supplementation strategy, should vitamin deficiency occur in patients undergoing orlistat therapy [14].

HIGHLIGHTS

Orlistat can be safely co-administred with the other drugs used for the treatment of patients with metabolic syndrome. However, highly lipophilic drugs could interact with orlistat and their absorption could be reduced.

References

[1] Drent ML, Larsson I, William-Olsson T, et al. Orlistat (Ro 18-0647), a lipase inhibitor, in the treatment of human obesity: a multiple dose study. *Int J Obes Relat Metab Disord.* 1995;19:221-226.

[2] Davidson MH, Hauptman J, DiGirolamo M, Foreyt JP, Halsted CH, Heber D, Heimburger DC, Lucas CP, Robbins DC, Chung J, Heymsfield SB Weight control and risk factor reduction in obese subjects treated for 2 years with orlistat: a randomized controlled trial. *JAMA*. 1999 Jan 20;281(3):235-42.

[3] Sjostrom L, Rissanen A, Andersen T, Boldrin M, Golay A, Koppeschaar HPF, Krempf M. Randomised placebo-controlled trial of orlistat for weight loss and prevention of weight regain in obese patients. *Lancet* 1998; 352: 167-172.

[4] O'Meara, S., Riemsma, R., Shirran, L., Mather, L. and ter Riet, G.A systematic review of the clinical effectiveness of orlistat used for the management of obesity. *Obesity Reviews* 5 (1), 51-68.

[5] Zhi J, Moore R, Kanitra L, Mulligan TE. Pharmacokinetic evaluation of the possible interaction between selected concomitant medications and orlistat at steady state in healthy subjects. *J Clin Pharmacol.* 2002 Sep;42(9):1011-9).

[6] Zhi J, Melia AT, Koss-Twardy SG, Min B, Guerciolini R, Freundlich NL, Milla G, Patel IHThe influence of orlistat on the pharmacokinetics and pharmacodynamics of glyburide in healthy volunteers. *J Clin Pharmacol.* 1995 May;35(5):521-5.

[7] Melia AT, Zhi J, Koss-Twardy SG, Min BH, Smith BL, Freundlich NL, Arora S, Passe SMThe influence of reduced dietary fat absorption induced by orlistat on the pharmacokinetics of digoxin in healthy volunteers. *J Clin Pharmacol.* 1995 Aug;35(8):840-3.

[8] Melia AT, Mulligan TE, Zhi J. Lack of effect of orlistat on the bioavailability of a single dose of nifedipine extended-release tablets (Procardia XL) in healthy volunteers. *J Clin Pharmacol.* 1996 Apr;36(4):352-5.

[9] Melia AT, Mulligan TE, Zhi J. The effect of orlistat on the pharmacokinetics of phenytoin in healthy volunteers. *J Clin Pharmacol.* 1996 Jul;36(7):654-8.

[10] Zhi J, Melia AT, Guerciolini R, Koss-Twardy SG, Passe SM, Rakhit A, Sadowski JAThe effect of orlistat on the pharmacokinetics and pharmacodynamics of warfarin in healthy volunteers. *J Clin Pharmacol.* 1996 Jul;36(7):659-66.)
[11] Melia AT, Zhi J, Zelasko R, Hartmann D, Guzelhan C, Guerciolini R, Odink J. The interaction of the lipase inhibitor orlistat with ethanol in healthy volunteers. *Eur J Clin Pharmacol.* 1998 Nov-Dec;54(9-10):773-7.
[12] Zhi J, Moore R, Kanitra L, Mulligan TE Effects of orlistat, a lipase inhibitor, on the pharmacokinetics of three highly lipophilic drugs (amiodarone, fluoxetine, and simvastatin) in healthy volunteers. *J Clin Pharmacol.* 2003 Apr;43(4):428-35.
[13] Zhi J, Moore R, Kanitra L, Mulligan TE. Pharmacokinetic evaluation of the possible interaction between selected concomitant medications and orlistat at steady state in healthy subjects. *J Clin Pharmacol.* 2002 Sep;42(9):1011-9.
[14] Melia AT, Koss-Twardy SG, Zhi J. The effect of orlistat, an inhibitor of dietary fat absorption, on the absorption of vitamins A and E in healthy volunteers. *J Clin Pharmacol.* 1996 Jul;36(7):647-53.

SIBUTRAMINE

Brief Compound Description

Sibutramine (Sibutramine hydrochloride monohydrate) is an orally administered. Its chemically the active ingredient is a racemic mixture of the (+) and (-) enantiomers of cyclobutanemethanamine 1-(4- chlorophenyl)-N, N - dimethyl - alfa - (2-methylpropyl)-, hydrochloride, monohydrate, and has an empirical formula of C17H 29Cl 2NO. Its molecular weight is 334.33. The structural formula of Sibutramine is the following:

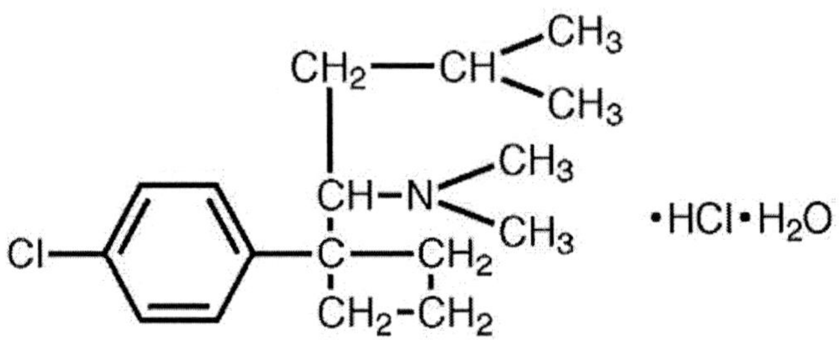

Mechanism of Action

Sibutramine inhibits reuptake and may stimulate release of the biogenic amine neurotransmitters dopamine, norepinephrine, and serotonin in the central nervous system (brain and spinal cord) and in the peripheral nervous system. Sibutramine increases the actions of these neurotransmitters. Sibutramine and its active metabolites are inhibitors of the reuptake of monoamines, primarily serotonin and noradrenaline and, to a lesser extent, dopamine. The pharmacologic effects of Sibutramine are mediated predominantly through its active primary (M1) and secondary (M2) amine metabolites,which are 100-fold more potent than the parent compound. Sibutramine is rapidly absorbed after oral administration; the time to peak plasma concentration (Tma x) is 1.2 hours. The drug undergoes extensive first-pass hepaticmetabolism by the cytochrome P-450 3A4 isozyme to form the active [1-8].

DRUG INTERACTIONS

Two categories of drug interactions are of concern: interactions based on the known mechanism of action of Sibutramine on biogenic amines, and interactions based on metabolism and elimination of Sibutramine. Main of the potential drug-drug interaction with Sibutramine are summarized in Table 1

Biogenic Amine Uptake Inhibition

Any drug that alters the function of dopamine, serotonin, or norepinephrine in the brain or peripheral nervous system has a strong potential for adverse interactions with Sibutramine (table 1).

Table 1. Potential drug-drug interactions with Sibutramine

SSRIs Fluoxetine,Fluvoxamine Paroxetine, Sertraline Venlafaxine
MAOIs Phenelzine, Selegiline
Opioids Dextromethorphan, Meperidine Pentazocine, Fentanyl Pethidine,
Antimigraine drugs Sumatriptan, Dihydroergotamine Others Lithium, Tryptophan
Ephedrine Pseudoephedrine
Cytochrome P-450 3A4 inhibitors Ketoconazole, Erythromycin Troleandomycin, Cyclosporine Grapefruit juice
Cytochrome P-450 3A4 inducers Rifampicin, Phenytoin Carbamazepine, Dexamethasone

SSRIs = selective serotonin reuptake inhibitors; MAOIs = monoamine oxidase inhibitors.

Metabolic Interactions

Sibutramine is metabolized primarily in the liver via the cytochrome oxidase P450 enzyme known as CYP 3A4. This pathway is remarkable because there is a substantial genetic heterogeneity in this enzyme that was determined by debrisoquine metabolism before the advent of molecule genetics.

HIGHLIGHTS

Sibutramine may interact with several medicines and cause a condition called Serotonin Syndrome. Do not prescribe sibutramine with other weight-loss products.

Main References

[1] P.E. Kaiser and J.L. Hinson, Sibutramine: Dose response and plasma metabolite concentrations in weight loss. *J Clin Pharmacol* 1994; 34:1019.

[2] C.J. Garratt, I.D. Hind and R.E. Haddock, Sibutramine metabolite bioavailability: Effect of dose level and food. *J Clin Pharmacol* 1995; 35: 927 Abstract.

[3] I.D. Hind, J.E. Mangham, S.P. Ghani et al., Sibutramine pharmacokinetics in young and elderly healthy subjects. *Eur J Clin Pharmacol* 1999 ;54: 847–849

[4] H.C. Jackson, M.C. Bearham, L.J. Hutchins et al., Investigation of the mechanisms underlying the hypophagic effects of the 5-HT and noradrenaline reuptake inhibitor, Sibutramine, in the rat. *Br J Pharmacol* 1997; 121; 1613–1618.

[5] S.C. Cheetham, J.A. Viggers, N.A. Slater et al., Inhibition of [3H]-paroxetine binding by Sibutramine, its metabolites and other antidepressants correlates with inhibition of [3H]-5-HT uptake. *Br J Pharmacol* 1990; 101; 515.

[6] C. Hanotin, F. Thomas, S.P. Jones et al., Efficacy and tolerability of Sibutramine in obese patients: A dose-ranging study. *Int J Obes Relat Metab Disord* 1998; 22: 32–38.

[7] G.A. Bray, D.H. Ryan, D. Gordon et al., A double-blind randomized placebo-controlled trial of Sibutramine. *Obes Res* 1996 ; 4: 263–270.

[8] M. Weintraub, A. Rubio, A. Golik et al., Sibutramine in weight control: A dose-ranging, efficacy study. *Clin Pharmacol Ther* 1991; 50: 330–337.

ENDOCANNABINOID RECEPTOR ANTAGONIST

The endocannabinoid system consists of several endogenous lipids, including anandamide and 2-arachidonoyl-glycerol (2-AG), and constitutes a retrograde signalling system, which modulates neurotransmitter release and synaptic plasticity. Specific brain-type cannabinoid receptors (CB(1)) are widely distributed in the central nervous system, and are localized presynaptically.

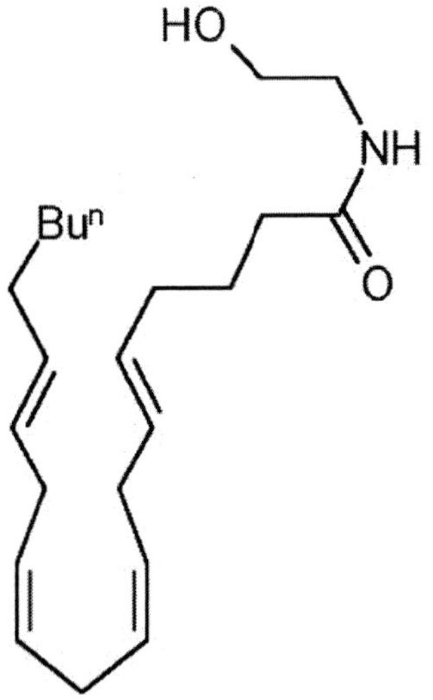

Structural formula of Anandamide

Growing evidences indicate that cannabinoids can act to increase food consumption, and cannabinoid CB [1] receptor antagonists/inverse agonists reduce food intake and suppress operant responding for food rewards. Hence, endocannabinoids provide the first example of a retrograde signalling system, which is strongly implicated in the control of food intake. Benzodiazepine and opioid palatability-dependent appetite are well-established processes supported by several sources of convergent evidence; they provide pharmacological benchmarks against which to evaluate the endocannabinoids. To date, evidence that endocannabinoids specifically modulate palatability as an affective evaluative process is insufficient and not compelling. Endocannabinoids may have important clinical utility in the treatment of human obesity and forms of eating disorders [1-3]. Anandamide is a prominent member of the endocannabinoids, a group of diffusible lipid molecules which influences neuronal excitability. In this context, endocannabinoids are known to modulate certain presynaptic Ca(2+) and K(+) channels, either through cannabinoid (CB1) receptor stimulation and second messenger pathway activation or by direct action [4].

RIMONABANT

Rimonabant is a selective CB1 endocannabinoid receptor antagonist indicated for the treatment of obesity. The drug, which has progressed to phase III development, works by blocking endogenous cannabinoid binding to neuronal CB1 receptors. Activation of these receptors by endoegenous cannabinoids, such as anadamide, increases appetite. It is the only endocannabinoid receptor antagonist in clinical development and thus offers a unique therapeutic approach to appetite control and weight reduction. The drug also has potential as a treatment for smoking cessation because the endocannabinoid system is also involved in the body's response to tobacco dependence. It could be brought to market in 2006 [5].

DRUG INTERACTIONS

Obviously, no data on the potential drug-drug interactions are still available from the literature.

Nevertheless, some very recent findings suggest that cyclooxygenase-2 (COX-2) limits endocannabinoid action. Hence there is growing interest on the pontential interactions with the anaesthetic agent propofol and the non-steroidal anti-inflammatory drugs indomethacin and flurbiprofen in activating cannabinoid receptors [6-7].

References

[1] Cooper SJ. Endocannabinoids and food consumption: comparisons with benzodiazepine and opioid palatability-dependent appetite.Eur J Pharmacol. 2004 Oct 1;500(1-3):37-49.

[2] Kirkham TC, Williams CM Endocannabinoid receptor antagonists: potential for obesity treatment. *Treat Endocrinol.* 2004;3(6):345-60.

[3] Di Marzo V, Goparaju SK, Wang L, Liu J, Batkai S, Jarai Z, Fezza F, Miura GI, Palmiter RD, Sugiura T, Kunos G. Leptin-regulated endocannabinoids are involved in maintaining food intake. *Nature.* 2001 Apr 12;410(6830):822-5.

[4] Nicholson RA, Liao C, Zheng J, David LS, Coyne L, Errington AC, Singh G, Lees G Sodium channel inhibition by anandamide and synthetic cannabimimetics in brain. *Brain Res.* 2003 Jul 18;978(1-2):194-204.

[5] Van Gaal LF, Rissanen A, Scheen A, Ziegler O, Rossner S.Effect of rimonabant on weight reduction and cardiovascular risk. Lancet. 2005 Jul 30-Aug 6;366(9483):369-70

[6] Kim J, Alger BE. Inhibition of cyclooxygenase-2 potentiates retrograde endocannabinoid effects in hippocampus. *Nat Neurosci.* 2004 Jul;7(7):697-8.

[7] Fowler CJ. Possible involvement of the endocannabinoid system in the actions of three clinically used drugs. *Trends Pharmacol Sci.* 2004 Feb;25(2):59-61.

Chapter 3

ORAL HYPOGLYCEMIC AND INSULIN SENSITIVE DRUGS

SULFONYLUREAS

General Drug Interactions

Sulfonylureas are partially or totally metabolised by the liver. The pharmacokinetics of the sulfonylureas subdived by generation are reported in *table 1*. Chlorpropamide is the only member of the class with substantial renal excretion, but is now rarely used. It is excreted much more rapidly in alkaline urine so its half-life and duration of action are reduced with excessive ingestion of alkalis. Antacids may increase the absorption of all the sulfonylureas and hence produce higher peak concentrations of the drugs and a risk of temporary hypoglycaemia. Sulfonylureas are highly protein bound drugs and may be displaced from blood protein binding sites by drugs such as the non-steroidal anti-inflammatory drugs. This can cause a short-term increase in free (unbound) sulfonylurea and hence temporary hypoglycaemia. The majority of significant interactions with sulfonylureas are due to the induction or inhibition of cytochrome P450 enzymes in the liver. The hypoglycemic action of sulfonylureas may be potentiated by certain drugs, including nonsteroidal anti-inflammatory drugs and other drugs that are highly protein bound, such as coumarins and beta adrenergic blocking agents. When these drugs are administered to a patient receiving sulfonylureas, the patient should be observed closely for hypoglycemia. When these drugs are withdrawn from a patient receiving sulfonylureas, the patient should be observed closely for loss of glycemic control. Certain drugs tend to produce hyperglycemia and may lead to loss of control. These drugs include the thiazides and other diuretics, corticosteroids, thyroid products, estrogens, oral contraceptives, nicotinic acid, sympathomimetics. When these drugs are administered to a patient receiving sulfonylureas, the patient should be closely observed for loss of control. When these drugs are withdrawn from a patient receiving sulfonylureas, the patient should be observed closely for hypoglycemia.

Table 1. Pharmacokinetics of the sulfonylureas

Generation	Generic Name	Metabolism	Renal Excretion of Active Metabolite
First	Chlorpropamide	Hepatic	Yes
First	Tolbutamide	Hepatic	Insignificant
First	Acetohexamide	Hepatic	Yes
First	Tolazamide	Hepatic	No
Second	Glipizide	Hepatic	No
Second	Glipizide	Hepatic	No
Second	Glyburide	Hepatic	Yes
Third	Glimepiride	Hepatic	Yes (?)

The main drug-drug interactions of first- and second-generation sulfonylureas are summarized in *Table 2.*

Table 2. Drug-drug interactions: first- and second-generation sulfonylureas.

Sulfonylurea	Drug	Mechanism	Effect
Chlorpropamide	Warfarin	⇓ Hepatic metabolism	Hypoglycemia
	Probenicid, allopurinol	⇓ Renal tubular secretion	Hypoglycemia
Tolbutamide	Digoxin		⇓ Digoxin level
	Warfarin	⇓ Hepatic metabolism	Hypoglycemia
Glipizide	Clofibrate	Displace from proteins	Hypoglycemia
	Cholestyramine	⇓ Absorption	Hypoglycemia
	H_2 blockers	⇓ Hepatic metabolism	Hypoglycemia
Glyburide	H_2 blockers	⇓ Hepatic metabolism	Hypoglycemia

Modified from Harrigan RA, et al. Oral agents for the treatment of type 2 diabetes mellitus: pharmacology, toxicity, and treatment. Ann Emerg Med. 2001 Jul;38(1):68-78.

Interactions between Sulphonylureas and KATP Channels Openers

ATP-sensitive potassium (KATP) channels are the targets for different classes of therapeutic drugs that are used in the treatment of diabetes, angina, and hypertension. The group of hypoglycaemic sulphonylureas and related drugs close KATP channels in pancreatic-cells, and thereby stimulate insulin release. The role of KATP channels under physiological conditions is to couple the electrical activity of cells to their metabolic rate. Under conditions when the metabolic rate is low, KATP channels are open, allowing K+ ions to pass out of the cell down their concentration gradient and thereby setting up a negative membrane potential. The metabolic rate of pancreatic -cells is modulated by the plasma glucose concentration. When the glucose level is low, -cells are hyperpolarised and do not release insulin. As the glucose concentration rises following a meal, the metabolic rate increases, KATP channels close, the membrane depolarises, voltage-gated Ca2+ channels open, and the influx of Ca2+ ions triggers insulin release [1]. The beta-cell K(ATP) channel is composed of two types of subunit - the inward rectifier K(+) channel (Kir6.2) which forms the channel pore, and the sulphonylurea receptor (SUR1), which serves as a regulatory subunit (Figure 1). Glibenclamide, tolbutamide and nateglinide binding appear to involve only SUR1 [2].

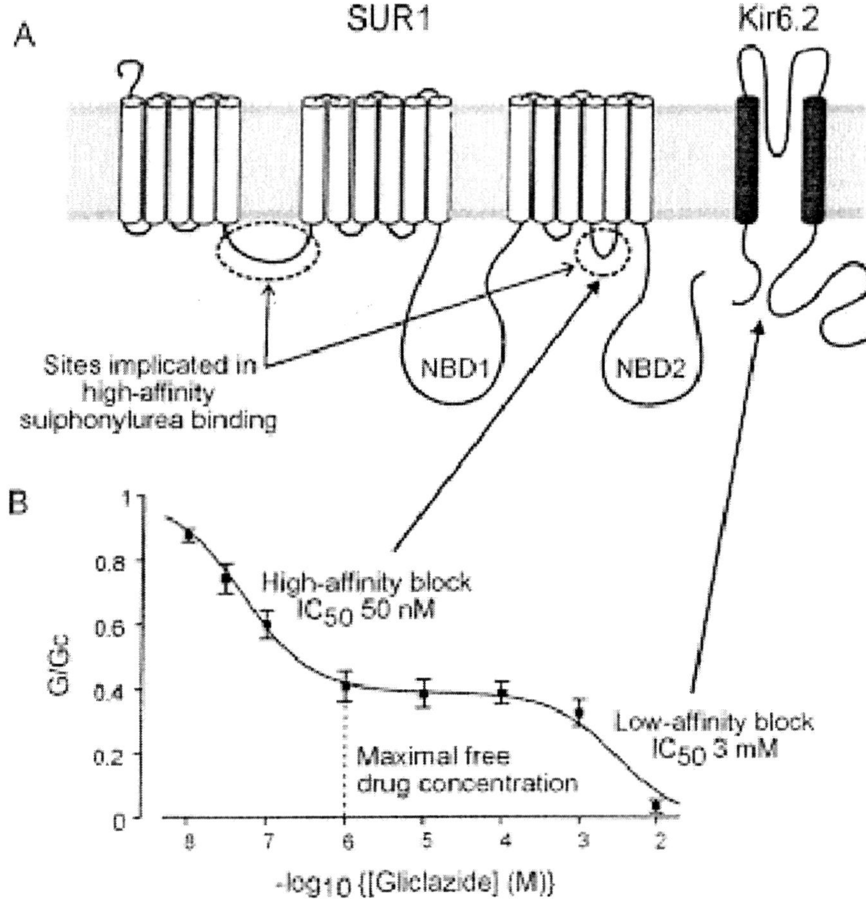

Figure 1. (A) Schematic representation of the membrane topology of Kir6.2 and sulphonylurea receptor subunits. NBD: nucleotide-binding domain. The locations of regions implicated in high-affinity binding of KATP channel inhibitors are indicated. (B) Dose–response curve for gliclazide block of Kir6.2/SUR1 and Kir6.2/SUR2A currents in Xenopus oocytes. The conductance in the presence of gliclazide (G) is expressed relative to that measured in control solution (Gc) High-affinity inhibition is mediated by the sulphonylurea receptor, whereas low-affinity block may involve direct drug interaction with Kir6.2. The maximum drug level measured in gliclazide-treated patients is indicated. (from Gribble and Ashcroft, 1999).

Drug Interactions

Sulphonylureas and KATP Channels Openers

Nicorandil, pinacidil, and diazoxide, by contrast, open KATP channels in vascular smooth muscle and cardiac muscle, cause muscle relaxation and vasodilation, and reduce myocardial work. The opposite actions of the two groups of drugs make it essential that clinically used therapeutic agents are tissue-specific.

Nicorandil is a new antianginal agent that potentially may be used to treat the cardiovascular side effects of diabetes. It is both a nitric oxide donor and an opener of ATP-sensitive K(+) (K(ATP)) channels in muscle and thereby causes vasodilation of the coronary vasculature. The antianginal agent nicorandil has a dual action on vascular smooth muscle, as it is both a KATP channel opener and a nitric oxide donor. Nicorandil activates KATP channels containing SUR2A or SUR2B by interaction with the C-terminal TM group of the SUR. The specificity for SUR2, exhibited by many KATP channel openers, has been attributed to sequence differences between SUR1 and SUR2 within this domain. Nevertheless, results about drug interaction between nicorandil and sulphonylureas are controversial. In fact, it has been reported that nicorandil activity was unaffected by gliclazide, which specifically blocks SUR1-type K(ATP) channels, but was severely impaired by glibenclamide and glimepiride, which target both SUR1 and SUR2-type K(ATP) channels [3]. By the contrast no antagonistic reactions from the combination of nicorandil with sulfonylurea have been described in patients with angina pectoris and diabetes mellitus [4].

References

[1] Ashcroft M. and Gribble, F.M. ATP-sensitive K+ channels and insulin secretion: their role in health and disease. *Diabetologia* 1999; 42: 903–919.

[2] Hansen AM, Hansen JB, Carr RD, Ashcroft FM, Wahl P. Kir6.2-dependent high-affinity repaglinide binding to beta-cell K(ATP) channels. *Br J Pharmacol.* 2005 Feb;144(4):551-7.

[3] Reimann F, Ashcroft FM, Gribble FM Structural basis for the interference between nicorandil and sulfonylurea action. *Diabetes*. 2001 Oct;50(10):2253-9.

[4] Hata N., Takano, M., Kunimi, H. and Takano, T. Lack of antagonism between nicorandil and sulfonylurea in stable angina pectoris. *International Journal of Clinical Pharmacology Research* 2001;321: 59–63.

GLYBURIDE (GLIBENCLAMIDE) AND GLIPIZIDE

Brief Compounds Description

The chemical name for glyburide is 1-[[*p* -[2-(5-chloro- *o* -anisamido)ethyl] phenyl]sulfonyl]-3-cyclohexyl-urea. The structural formula is represented below:

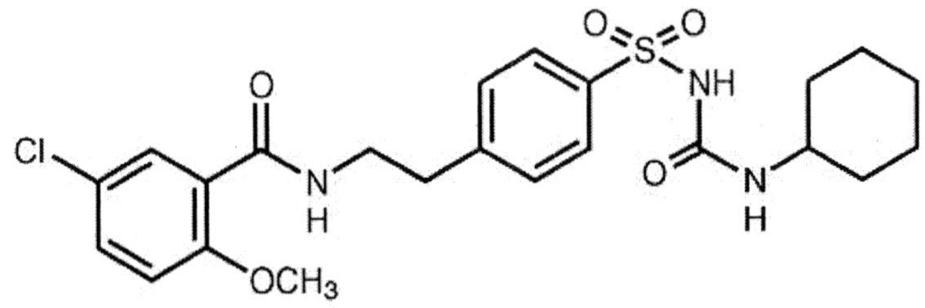

Glyburide

The chemical name of glipizide is 1-cyclohexyl-3-[[p-[2-(5-methylpyrazine-carboxamido)ethyl] phenyl]sulfonyl]urea. The molecular formula is $C_{21}H_{27}N_5O_4S$; the molecular weight is 445.55; the structural formula is shown below:

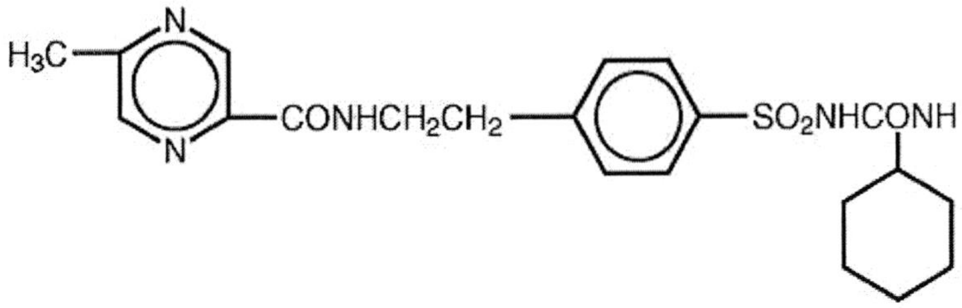

Drug Interaction Mechanisms

The inhibitory effect of glyburide on CYP1A2, CYP2C8, CYP2C9, CYP2C19, CYP2D6, CYP2E1, and CYP3A4 activities was evaluated using pooled human liver microsomes. Glyburide showed potent inhibition on CYP2C9 and weak inhibition on CYP3A4, whereas it had minimal or no inhibitory effect on the other cytochromes p450 examined. It is anticipated that clinically significant drug-drug interactions will ensue when glyburide is coadministered with agents that are cleared primarily by the CYP2C9-mediated pathway and those with narrow therapeutic ranges [1].

Drug Interactions

Glyburide is reported to cause drug interactions with numerous drugs leading to an increase or decrease in the glyburide concentration, resulting in hypoglycemia or hyperglycemia. Conversely, several studies have shown that glyburide inhibited coadministered drugs [2]. Some of the drug interactions them are detailed below.

Glibenclamide and H2-Receptor Antagonists

Plasma glucose concentrations were unexpectedly higher when glibenclamide was administered with cimetidine or ranitidine when compared with glibenclamide administered alone. Plasma insulin concentrations were significantly elevated when H2-receptor antagonists and glibenclamide were administered concurrently [3].

Glyburide and Bosentan

The plasma levels of both bosentan and glyburide were reduced after concomitant administration. This finding is consistent with a CYP3A4-inducing potential of both drugs. The observed pharmacodynamic interaction between bosentan and glyburide in patients with chronic heart failure cannot be explained by a pharmacokinetic interaction [4].

References

[1] Kim KA, Park JY Inhibitory effect of glyburide on human cytochrome p450 isoforms in human liver microsomes. *Drug Metab Dispos.* 2003 Sep;31(9):1090-2.

[2] Asplund K, Wiholm BE, and Lithner F Glibenclamide-associated hypoglycaemia: a report on 57 cases. *Diabetologia* 1983; 24: 412-417.

[3] Kubacka RT, Antal EJ, Juhl RP. The paradoxical effect of cimetidine and ranitidine on glibenclamide pharmacokinetics and pharmacodynamics. *Br J Clin Pharmacol* 1987; 23: 743-751.

[4] van Giersbergen PL, Treiber A, Clozel M, Bodin F, Dingemanse J In vivo and in vitro studies exploring the pharmacokinetic interaction between bosentan, a dual endothelin receptor antagonist, and glyburide. *Clin Pharmacol Ther.* 2002 Apr;71(4):253-62.

GLIMEPIRIDE

Brief Compound Description

Glimepiride is an oral blood-glucose-lowering drug of the sulfonylurea class Chemically, glimepiride is identified as 1-[[p-[2-(3-ethyl-4-methyl-2-oxo-3-pyrroline-1-carboxamido) ethyl]phenyl]sulfonyl]-3-(trans-4methylcyclohexyl)urea.The structural formula is the following:

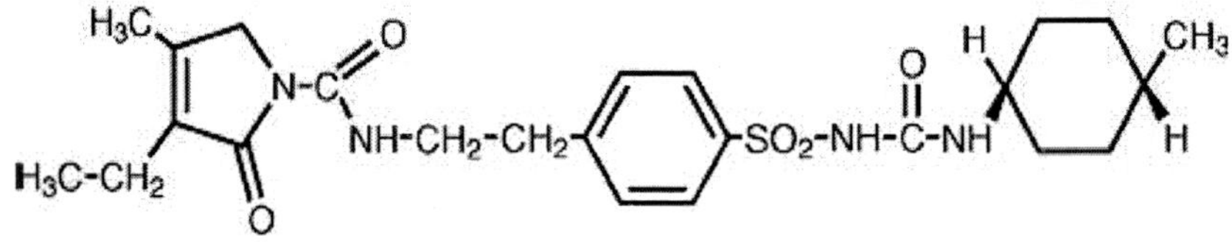

Mechanism of Action

The primary mechanism of action of glimepiride in lowering blood glucose appears to be dependent on stimulating the release of insulin from functioning pancreatic beta cells. In addition, extrapancreatic effects may also play a role in the activity of sulfonylureas such as glimepiride.

Drug Interactions

Main of the potential drug-drug interaction with Glimepiride during treatment of metabolic syndrome are summarized in Table 1. Some of them are detailed below.

Table 1. Potential drug interactions with glimepiride in metabolic syndrome

NO	Potential
Aspirin	Beta-blockers
Beta-blockers	
Warfarin,	Diclofenac, Ibuprofen, Naproxen
ACE inhibitor	
Calcium-channel blockers,	
Estrogens	
Fibrates, HMG CoA reductase inhibitors	
Thyroid hormone	

Glimepiride and Aspirin

Coadministration of aspirin and glimepiride led to a 34% decrease in the mean glimepiride AUC. The mean Cmax had a decrease of 4%. Blood glucose and serum C-peptide concentrations were unaffected and no hypoglycemic symptoms were reported. Data from clinical trials showed no evidence of clinically significant adverse interactions with uncontrolled concurrent administration of aspirin and other salicylates.

Glimepiride and Propranolol

Concomitant administration of propranolol (40 mg day) and glimepiride significantly increased Cmax, AUC, and T1/2 of glimepiride by 23%, 22%, and 15%, respectively, and it decreased CL/f by 18%. The pharmacodynamic responses to glimepiride were nearly identical in normal subjects receiving propranolol and placebo. Data from clinical trials in patients with type 2 diabetes showed no evidence of clinically significant adverse interactions with uncontrolled concurrent administration of beta-blockers. However, if beta-blockers are used, caution should be exercised and patients should be warned about the potential for hypoglycemia.

Glimepiride and Warfarin

Concomitant administration of glimepiride tablets (4 mg once daily) did not alter the pharmacokinetic characteristics of R- and S-warfarin enantiomers following administration of a single dose (25 mg) of racemic warfarin to healthy subjects. No changes were observed in warfarin plasma protein binding. glimepiride treatment did result in a slight, but statistically significant, decrease in the pharmacodynamic response to warfarin. The reductions in mean area under the prothrombin time (PT) curve and maximum PT values during glimepiride treatment were very small (3.3% and 9.9%, respectively) and are unlikely to be clinically important.

Glimepiride and Ramipril

The responses of serum glucose, insulin, C-peptide, and plasma glucagon to 2 mg glimepiride were unaffected by coadministration of ramipril 5 mg once daily in normal subjects. No hypoglycemic symptoms were reported. Data from clinical trials in patients with NIDDM showed no evidence of clinically significant adverse interactions with uncontrolled concurrent administration of ACE inhibitors.

Glimepiride and Calcium-channel Blockers, Estrogens, Fibrates, NSAIDS, HMG CoA Reductase Inhibitors, Thyroid Hormone

Although no specific interaction studies were performed, pooled data from clinical trials showed no evidence of clinically significant adverse interactions with uncontrolled concurrent administration of calcium-channel blockers, estrogens, fibrates, NSAIDS, HMG CoA reductase inhibitors, or thyroid hormone.

Glimepiride and Cimetidine

Coadministration of either cimetidine (800 mg once daily) or ranitidine (150 mg bid) with a single 4-mg oral dose of glimepiride did not significantly alter the absorption and disposition of glimepiride, and no differences were seen in hypoglycemic symptomatology. Pooled data from clinical trials showed no evidence of clinically significant adverse interactions with uncontrolled concurrent administration of H2-receptor antagonists.

HIGHLIGHTS

Glimepiride can be safely co-administred with the other drugs used for the treatment of patients with metabolic syndrome. However, the concomitant use of glimepiride and beta-blockers should be exercised with caution

MEGLITINIDES

Repaglinide

Brief Compound Description

Repaglinide, S(+) 2-ethoxy-4(2((3-methyl-1-(2-(1-piperidinyl) phenyl)-butyl)amino)-2-oxoethyl) benzoic acid, is chemically unrelated to the oral sulfonylurea insulin secretagogues. The structural formula is as shown below:

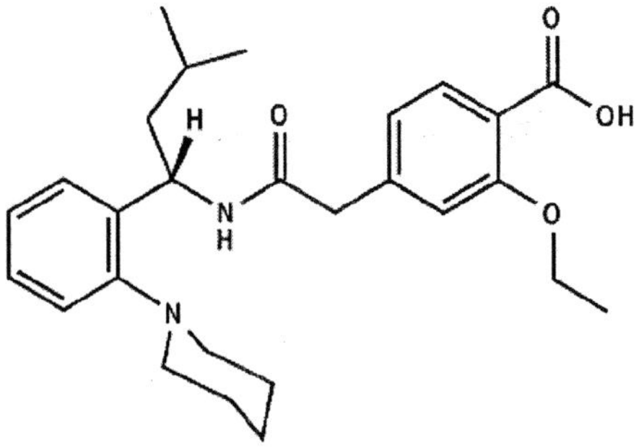

Mechanism of Action

Repaglinide is a short-acting meglitinide analog antidiabetic drug. Although repaglinide binds to the sulphonylurea binding sites on pancreatic beta-cells and has a similar mechanism of action, repaglinide exhibits distinct pharmacological properties compared with these agents. Following administration, repaglinide is absorbed rapidly and has a fast onset of dose-dependent blood-glucose lowering effect. The drug is eliminated rapidly via the biliary route, without accumulation in the plasma after multiple doses.

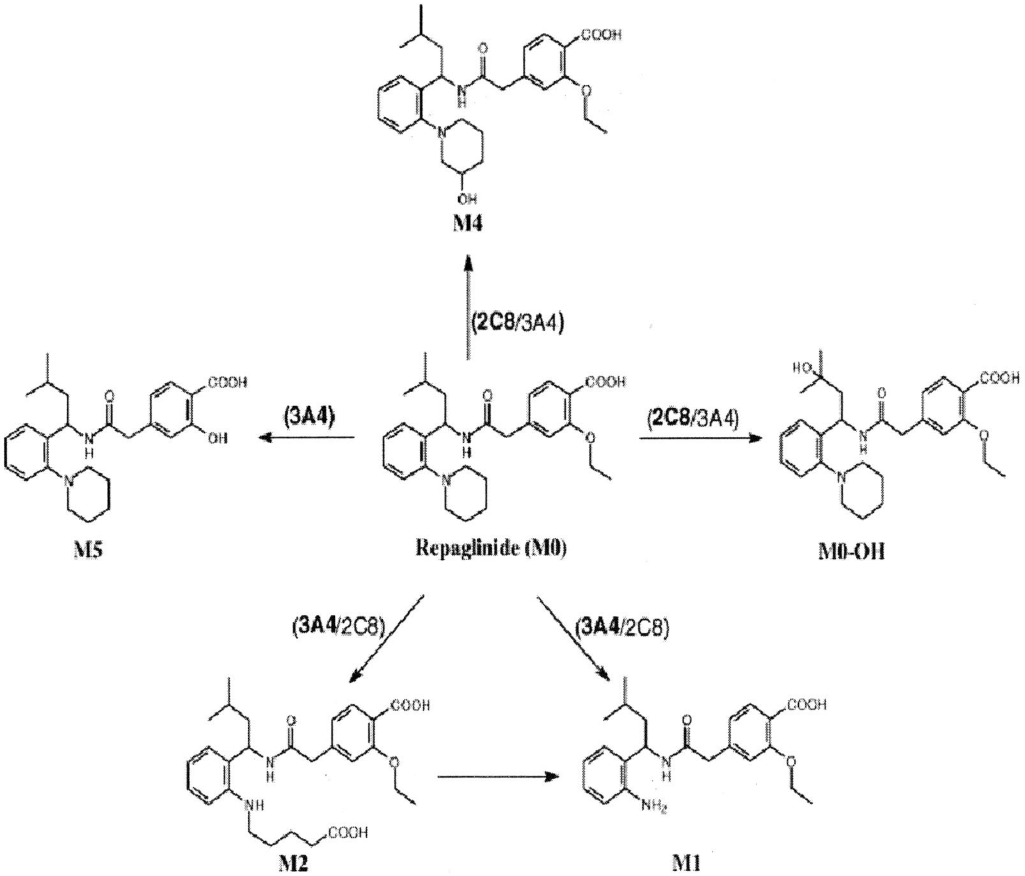

M4

(2C8/3A4)

M5 (3A4) Repaglinide (M0) (2C8/3A4) M0-OH

(3A4/2C8) (3A4/2C8)

M2 M1

Figure. Biotransformation pathways of repaglinide in vitro. The principal enzyme responsible is highlighted in bold.

Repaglinide is metabolized mainly by CYP2C8 and CYP3A4. Variation in the activities of these enzymes may lead to a better understanding of the difference in AUC and C max observed within patient groups treated with repaglinide. Metabolism by both these enzymes may also explain why selective inhibition and possibly induction of CYP3A4 in humans has a less than expected effect on repaglinide pharmacokinetics and effect [2].

Drug Interactions

Drug interaction studies were carried out to ensure that hypoglycemia due to inhibition of repaglinide elimination or chronic hyperglycemia due to inhibition of repaglinide absorption was avoided. Main of the potential drug-drug interaction with Repaglinide in the context of metabolic syndrome are summarized in Table 1. Some of these are discussed in detail below. Other potential interactions between repaglinide and drugs which alter hepatic enzymes are reported in Table 2.

Table 1. Potential drug-drug interactions with Repaglinide in metabolic syndrome

YES	Mechanism and effect	NO
Gemfibrozil	⇒ prolonged blood glucose-lowering effect of repaglinide	Digoxin Bezafibrate, Fenofibrate Simvastatin Ethinyloestradiol/ Levonorgestrel Nifedipine

Repaniglinide and Gemfibrozil

Gemfibrozil raised the area under the plasma concentration-time curve (AUC) of repaglinide 8.1-fold and prolonged its half-life (t1/2). Gemfibrozil considerably enhanced and prolonged the blood glucose-lowering effect of repaglinide. Potentially hazardous interaction between gemfibrozil and repaglinide could occur. Concomitant use of gemfibrozil and repaglinide should be best avoided. If the combination is considered necessary, repaglinide dosage should be greatly reduced and blood glucose concentrations carefully monitored [3].

Repaglinide and Bezafibrate and Fenofibrate

Bezafibrate and fenofibrate had no significant effect on the peak concentration (Cmax) of repaglinide. The blood glucose-lowering effect of repaglinide was not affected by bezafibrate or fenofibrate. Neither bezafibrate nor fenofibrate affected the pharmacokinetic variables of repaglinide. Bezafibrate and fenofibrate do not affect the pharmacokinetics or pharmacodynamics of repaglinide [4].

Repaglinide and Ethinyloestradiol/levonorgestrel, Simvastatin, and Nifedipine

Drug interactions between repaglinide and other drugs interacting with CYP3A4: ethinyloestradiol/levonorgestrel, simvastatin, and nifedipine have been analyzed. No clinically relevant pharmacokinetic interactions occurred between repaglinide and the CYP3A4 substrates ethinyloestradiol/levonorgestrel, simvastatin, or nifedipine.. No safety concerns were observed, except a higher incidence in adverse events in patients receiving repaglinide and simvastatin or nifedipine [5].

Repaglinide and Digoxin

The coadministration of repaglinide and digoxin did not influence the pharmacokinetics of digoxin administered alone. No direct drug-drug interactions were found in these studies, suggesting that repaglinide may be coprescribed with digoxin at the dosage used for monotherapy [6].

Repaglinide and Grapefruit Juice

Grapefruit juice interacting with the antidiabetic agent repaglinide may cause hypoglycemia [7].

HIGHLIGHTS

Repaglinide can be safely co-administred with the majority of the drugs used for the treatment of patients with metabolic syndrome. However, a potential interaction between repaglinide and gemfibrozil hsas been described and the blood glucose-lowering effect of repaglinide could be prolonged. By the contrast, neither bezafibrate nor fenofibrate affect the pharmacokinetics or pharmacodynamics of repaglinide

REFERENCES

[1] Hatorp, V., Clinical pharmacokinetics and pharmacodynamics of repaglinide. *Clin Pharmacokinet* 2002 ; 41: 471–483.

[2] Bidstrup TB, Bjornsdottir I, Sidelmann UG, Thomsen MS, Hansen KTCYP2C8 and CYP3A4 are the principal enzymes involved in the human in vitro biotransformation of the insulin secretagogue repaglinide. *Br J Clin Pharmacol.* 2003 Sep;56(3):305-14.

[3] Niemi, J.T. Backman, M. Neuvonen and P.J. Neuvonen, Effects of gemfibrozil, itraconazole, and their combination on the pharmacokinetics and pharmacodynamics of repaglinide: potentially hazardous interaction between gemfibrozil and repaglinide. *Diabetologia* 46 (2003), pp. 347–351.

[4] Kajosaari LI, Backman JT, Neuvonen M, Laitila J, Neuvonen PJ. Lack of effect of bezafibrate and fenofibrate on the pharmacokinetics and pharmacodynamics of repaglinide. *Br J Clin Pharmacol.* 2004 Oct;58(4):390-6.

[5] Hatorp V, Hansen KT, Thomsen MS Influence of drugs interacting with CYP3A4 on the pharmacokinetics, pharmacodynamics, and safety of the prandial glucose regulator repaglinide. *J Clin Pharmacol.* 2003 Jun;43(6):649-60.

[6] Hatorp V, Thomsen MS Drug interaction studies with repaglinide: repaglinide on digoxin or theophylline pharmacokinetics and cimetidine on repaglinide pharmacokinetics. *J Clin Pharmacol.* 2000 Feb;40(2):184-92.

[7] Bailey DG, Dresser GKInteractions between grapefruit juice and cardiovascular drugs. *Am J Cardiovasc Drugs.* 2004;4(5):281-97.

NATEGLINIDE

Brief Compound Description

Nateglinide, N-[trans-4-isopropylcyclohexane)carbonyl]-D-phenylalanine, is structurally unrelated to the oral sulfonylurea insulin secretagogues. The structural formula is as shown below:

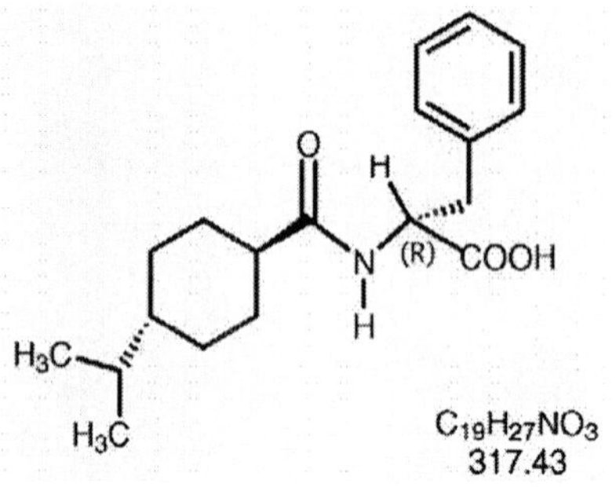

$C_{19}H_{27}NO_3$
317.43

Mechanism of Action

Nateglinide is a phenylalanine derivative that blocks K+ channels in pancreatic beta-cells, facilitating insulin secretion. Nateglinide sensitises beta-cells to ambient glucose, reducing the glucose concentration needed to stimulate insulin secretion. The pharmacokinetics of nateglinide are characterised by rapid absorption and elimination, with good bioavailability. Nateglinide is more rapidly absorbed when given 0-30 minutes prior to meal ingestion than if given during the meal. Nateglinide is extensively metabolised, primarily by cytochrome P450 2C9, and eliminated primarily by the kidney. No significant pharmacokinetic alterations occur in renally impaired patients, in the elderly, or in mildly hepatically impaired patients [1].

Drug Interactions

Nateglinide and Warfarin

The concurrent administration of nateglinide and warfarin did not affect the maximal change in prothrombin time that follows warfarin administration. No effect of coadministration of nateglinide on the pharmacodynamic action of warfarin or any pharmacokinetic interactions between warfarin and nateglinide have been reported [2].

Nateglinide and Acenocoumarol

Co-administration of nateglinide does not influence either the pharmacokinetics or the anticoagulant activity of R- and S-acenocoumarol in healthy subjects. This suggests that no dosage adjustments will be required when nateglinide and acenocoumarol are coadministered in clinical practice [3].

Main References

[1] McLeod JF Clinical pharmacokinetics of nateglinide: a rapidly-absorbed, short-acting insulinotropic agent. *Clin Pharmacokinet.* 2004;43(2):97-120.

[2] Anderson DM, Shelley S, Crick N, Buraglio M No effect of the novel antidiabetic agent nateglinide on the pharmacokinetics and anticoagulant properties of warfarin in healthy volunteeers. *J Clin Pharmacol.* 2002 Dec;42(12):1358-65.

[3] Sunkara G, Bigler H, Wang Y, Smith H, Prasad P, McLeod J, Ligueros-Saylan M The effect of nateglinide on the pharmacokinetics and pharmacodynamics of acenocoumarol. *Curr Med Res Opin.* 2004 Jan;20(1):41-8.

METFORMIN

Brief Compound Description

Metformin (N,N-dimethylimidodicarbonimidic diamide hydrochloride) is a compound with a molecular formula of C4H11N5 • HCl and a molecular weight of 165.63. Metformin hydrochloride is freely soluble in water and is insoluble in acetone, ether, and chloroform. The structural formula of Metformin is the following:

$$(H_3C)_2N-\underset{\|}{C}(=NH)-NH-\underset{\|}{C}(=NH)-NH_2 \cdot HCl$$

Main Mechanisms of Action

Metformin is the only available biguanide (dimethyl-biguanide) [2]. Metformin is an oral antidiabetic drug, which decreased hepatic glucose output due to decreased hepatic gluconeogenesis and increased glycogenesis and lipogenesis, decreases intestinal absorption of glucose and improves insulin sensitivity by increasing peripheral glucose uptake and utilization [3-6]. The way of metformin administration affects the kinetics and extent of its pharmacological action [7]. In fact, it has been reported that a bolus peroral administration of the drug produced stronger and longer glucose-lowering response than i.v. administration of an equivalent dose [7]. Differences in the infusion site have been also described. The major difference between infusion of metformin to the duodenum and the peripheral vein is the targeting of higher drug concentrations to presystemic biophases over a prolonged period of time. Intraduodenal bolus and infusion produced higher portal-vein metformin concentrations and thereby enhanced exposure of the liver/portal biophase to metformin compared with i.v.

infusions. Gastrointestinal administration of metformin, in addition to elevated portal exposure, leads also to higher exposure of the gastrointestinal biophase to the drug [8].

Drug Interactions

Main of the possible drug-drug interactions between Metformin and other components used in patients with metabolic syndrome are summarized in Table 1. Some of these potential interactions are discussed in detail below.

Table 1. Potential drug-drug interactions with Metformin in metabolic syndrome

YES	Potential	Mechanism	NO	Unclear
Furosemide	Amiloride Triamterene	⇑ increased concentration of metformin	Sulfonylureas	Orlistat
			Atenolol	
Nifedipine	Verapamil Diltiazem Felodipine Amlodipine	⇑ increased concentration of metformin		
		⇑ increased concentration of metformin		
Cimetidine Ranitidine				
	Digoxin, Procainamide Quinidine	⇑ increased concentration of metformin		

Metformin and Glyburide

In a single-dose interaction study in type 2 diabetes patients, co-administration of metformin and glyburide did not result in any changes in either metformin pharmacokinetics or pharmacodynamics. Decreases in glyburide AUC and Cmax were observed, but were highly variable.The single-dose nature of this study and the lack of correlation between glyburide blood levels and pharmacodynamic effects, makes the clinical significance of this interaction uncertain

Metformin and Furosemide

A single-dose, metformin-furosemide drug interaction study in healthy subjects demonstrated that pharmacokinetic parameters of both compounds were affected by coadministration. Furosemide increased the metformin plasma and blood Cmax by 22% and blood. AUC by 15%, without any significant change in metformin renal clearance. When administered with metformin, the Cmax and AUC of furosemide were 31% and 12% smaller, respectively, than when administered alone, and the terminal half-life was decreased by 32%, without any significant change in furosemide renal clearance. No information is available about the interaction of metformin and furosemide when co-administered chronically.

Metformin and Nifedipine

A single-dose, metformin-nifedipine drug interaction study in normal healthy volunteers demonsrated that co-administration of nifedipine increased plasma metformin Cmax and AUC by 20% and 9%, respectively, and increased the amount excreted in the urine. Tmax and half-life were unaffected. Nifedipine appears to enhance the absorption of metformin. Metformin had minimal effects on nifedipine.

Metformin and Cationic Drugs

Metformin and Cationic drugs (amiloride, digoxin, morphine, procainamide, quinidine, ranitidine, triamterene) that are eliminated by renal tubular secretion theoretically have the potential for interaction with metformin by competing for common renal tubular transport systems. Although such interactions remain theoretical, careful patient monitoring and dose adjustment of Metformin and/or the interfering drug is recommended in patients who are taking cationic medications that are excreted via the proximal renal tubular secretory system.

Metformin and Cimetidine

Such interaction between metformin and oral cimetidine has been observed in normal healthy volunteers in both single- and multiple-dose, metformin-cimetidine drug interaction studies, with a 60% increase in peak metformin plasma and whole blood concentrations and a 40% increase in plasma and whole blood metformin AUC. There was no change in elimination half-life in the single-dose study. Metformin had no effect on cimetidine pharmacokinetics. [9].

Metformin and Atenolol

Treatment with atenolol alone does not significantly change metformin levels, however administration of metformin or atenolol/metformin increased significantly the glutathione (GSH) levels in both liver and blood, and returned the liver Mg content back to normal values [10].

Metformin and Orlistast

The pharmacokinetic interactions of orlistat, a pancreatic lipase inhibitor that reduces intestinal absorbtion of dietary fat by up to 37% [8], have only recently been explored [11-13], but no interactions between orlistat and metformin have been reported. Nevertheless, a possible metformin and orlistast interaction in inducing lactic acidosis has been hypothesized. Orlistat could have played a role in the development of lactic acidosis in patients who are taking metformin by some potential mechanisms.

Metformin and Rofecoxib

Rofecoxib may have been a precipitating factor of metformin-induced lactic acidosis. The risk of renal failure with the use of traditional NSAIDs is well known. What is less well appreciated is the role that the COX 2 inhibitors may play in the development of renal failure which, when it occurs in a patient on metformin, can lead to a potentially disastrous outcome [14].

HIGHLIGHTS

Metformin can be safely co-administred with the majority of the drugs used for the treatment of patients with metabolic syndrome. However, some potential interactions between metformin and cationic drugs and calcium channels blockers have been reported.

REFERENCES

[1] Metformin extended release--DepoMed: metformin, metformin gastric retention, metformin GR. *Drugs R D.* 2004;5(4):231-3.

[2] Bailey C, Path M, Turner R (1996) Drug therapy: metformin. New England Journal of Medicine, 334, 574–579.

[3] Hermann L and Melander A (1992) Biguanides: basic aspects and clinical uses, in *International Textbook of Diabetes Mellitus* (Alberti KGMM, DeFronzo RA, Keen H and Zimmet P eds) John Wiley and Sons Inc., New York.

[4] Cusi K,DeFronzo RA Metformin: a review of its metabolic effects. *Diab Rev* 1998;6:89-13.

[5] Christiansen MP and Hellerstein MK Effects of metformin on hepatic glucose metabolism. *Curr Opin Endocrinol Diabetes* 1998; 5: 252-255.

[6] Wilcock C and Bailey CJ Reconsideration of inhibitory effect of metformin on intestinal glucose absorption. *J Pharm Pharmacol* 1991; 43: 120-121.

[7] Stepensky D, Friedman M, Raz I, Hoffman A Pharmacokinetic-pharmacodynamic analysis of the glucose-lowering effect of metformin in diabetic rats reveals first-pass pharmacodynamic effect. *Drug Metab Dispos.* 2002 Aug;30(8):861-8.

[8] Hoffman A and Stepensky D. Pharmacodynamic aspects of modes of drug administration for optimization of drug therapy. *Crit Rev Ther Drug Carrier Syst* 1999; 16: 571-639.

[9] Somogyi A, Stockley C, Keal J, Rolan P, Bochner F Reduction of metformin renal tubular secretion by cimetidine in man. *Br J Clin Pharmacol.* 1987 May;23(5):545-51

[10] 10 Ewis SA, Abdel-Rahman MS. Influence of atenolol and/or metformin on glutathione and magnesium levels in diabetic rats. *J Appl Toxicol.* 1997 Nov-Dec;17(6):409-13.

[11] Sjostrom L, Rissanen A, Andersen T et al: Randomised placebo-controlled trial of orlistat for weight loss and prevention of weight regain in obese patients: European Multicentre Orlistat Study Group. *Lancet* 352:167–172, 1998.

[12] Dawson D, Conlon C. Case study: metformin-associated lactic acidosis: could orlistat be relevant? *Diabetes Care.* 2003 Aug;26(8):2471-2.

[13] Zhi J, Moore R, Kanitra L, Mulligan TE: Pharmacokinetic evaluation of the possible interaction between selected concomitant medications and orlistat at steady state in healthy subjects. *J Clin Pharmacol* 42:1011–1019, 2002.

[14] Price G. Metformin lactic acidosis, acute renal failure and rofecoxib. *Br J Anaesth.* 2003 Dec;91(6):909-10.

THIAZOLIDINEDIONES (GLITAZONES)

Mechanisms of Action

Thiazolidinediones (TZDs) form a new class of oral antidiabetic agents. They improve insulin sensitivity and reduce glycemia, lipidemia and insulinemia in patients with type 2 diabetes. They activate the nuclear receptor Peroxisome Proliferator-Activated Receptor gamma (PPARgamma), altering the expression of genes involved in glucose and lipid homeostasis. Stimulating PPARgamma improves insulin sensitivity via several mechanisms: 1) it raises the expression of GLUT4 glucose transporter; 2) it regulates release of adipocyte-derived signaling factors that affect insulin sensitivity in muscle, and 3) it contributes to a turn-over in adipose tissue, inducing the production of smaller, more insulin sensitive adipocytes. Clinically TZDs improves sensitivity to insulin in muscle and adipose tissue and inhibits hepatic gluconeogenesis. TZDs also affect free fatty acids lipotoxicity on islets, improving pancreatic B-cell function. In addition, triglycerides and FFA levels are lowered by TZDs. As for side effects, rosiglitazone and pioglitazone may cause increased plasma volume, edema and dose-related weight gain. TZDs offer an attractive option in the treatment of type 2 diabetes, though it may be too soon to determine if they prevent vascular complications, as do other oral antidiabetic agents. An important issue for the future will be to assess the influence of weight gain in the long time [1-4].

Drug Interactions Mechanisms

Thiazolidinediones, rosiglitazone and pioglitazone, have been reported to induce cytochrome P450 enzymes (P450) in primary human hepatocyte cultures and to inhibit P450 in human microsomes [5-6]. Troglitazone was withdrawn from the market on 2000. Rosiglitazone and pioglitazone have the potential to induce CYP3A4, and the resulting clinical outcome of the CYP3A4 induction may be related to the dose and subsequent pharmacokinetics of each drug. The oxidative metabolism of pioglitazone is through CYP3A4 and CYP2C8, whereas rosiglitazone is metabolized by CYP2C8 and to a minor extent by CYP2C9 Nevertheless the data in this area are quite controversial. In fact, some data indicate that at the doses administered, rosiglitazone and pioglitazone are not significant inducers or inhibitors of CYP3A4 or CYP2C9 [7].

Thiazolidinedione and Statins

The exact mechanism for the statin-thiazolidinedione interaction is not well defined and controversial results have been reported. The thiazolidinediones exert their therapeutic effect by activating the peroxisome proliferator-activated receptor. It has been suggested that the peroxisome proliferator- activated receptor family may modulate the function of the cytochrome P450 system. This influence on cytochrome P450 function raises concerns regarding potential drug–drug interactions between the thiazolidinediones and simvastatin or atorvastatin, which are significantly metabolized through the cytochrome P450-3A4 system

Main References

[1] Dubois M, Vantyghem MC, Schoonjans K, Pattou F. Thiazolidinediones in type 2 diabetes. Role of peroxisome proliferator-activated receptor gamma (PPARgamma] *Ann Endocrinol* (Paris). 2002 Dec;63(6 Pt 1):511-23.

[2] Schoonjans K, Auwerx J Thiazolidinediones: an update. *Lancet.* 2000 Mar 18;355(9208):1008-10

[3] Stumvoll M, Haring HU Glitazones: clinical effects and molecular mechanisms. *Ann Med.* 2002;34(3):217-24

[4] Yki-Jarvinen H, Thiazolidinediones. N. *Engl. J. Med.,* September 9, 2004; 351(11): 1106 – 1118.

[5] Sahi J, Black CB, Hamilton GA, Zheng X, Jolley S, Rose KA, Gilbert D, LeCluyse EL, Sinz MW. Comparative effects of thiazolidinediones on in vitro P450 enzyme induction and inhibition. *Drug Metab Dispos.* 2003 Apr;31(4):439-46.

[6] Yamazaki H, Suzuki M, Tane K, Shimadi N, Nakajima M and Yokoi T (2000) In vitro inhibitory effects of troglitazone and its metabolites on drug oxidation activities of human cytochrome P450 enzymes: comparison with pioglitazone and rosiglitazone. *Xenobiotica* 30: 61-70.

[7] Loi C, Young M, Randinitis E, Vassos A, Koup J. Clinical pharmacokinetics of troglitazone. *Clin Pharmacokinet* 1999; 37: 91-104.

ROSIGLITAZONE

Brief Compound Description

Chemically,rosiglitazone maleate is (±)-5-[[4-[2-(methyl-2 pyridinylamino)ethoxy] phenyl]methyl]-2,4-thiazolidinedione, (Z)-2-butenedioate (1:1) with a molecular weight of 473.52 (357.44 free base). The molecule has a single chiral center and is present as a racemate. The structural formula of rosiglitazone maleate is: The molecular formula is C18H19N3O3S•C4H4O4. Structural formula of Rosiglitazone is the following:

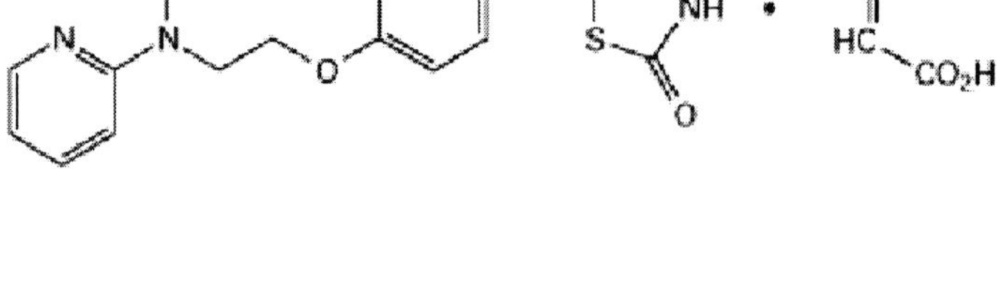

Drug Interactions

Main of the possible drug-drug interactions between rosiglitazone and other components used in patients with metabolic syndrome are summarized in Table 1. Some of these potential interactions are discussed in detail below.

Table 1. Potential drug-drug interactions with rosiglitazone in metabolic syndrome

YES	Mechanism	NO
Gemfibrozil	⇑ increased concentration of rosiglitazone	Acarbose Digoxin Nifedipine
		Oral contraceptives Ranitidine Sucralfate

Drugs that Inhibit, Induce, or are Metabolized by Cytochrome P450

In vitro drug metabolism studies suggest that rosiglitazone does not inhibit any of the major P450 enzymes at clinically relevant concentrations. In vitro data demonstrate that rosiglitazone is predominantly metabolized by CYP2C8, and to a lesser extent, 2C9.

Drug Interactions: An Inhibitor of CYP2C8

Drug Interactions: An inhibitor of CYP2C8 (such as gemfibrozil) may increase the AUC of rosiglitazone and an inducer of CYP2C8 may decrease the AUC of rosiglitazone. Therefore, if an inhibitor or an inducer of CYP2C8 is started or stopped during treatment with rosiglitazone, changes in diabetes treatment may be needed based upon clinical response.

Rosiglitazone and Gemfibrozil

Co-administration of gemfibrozil (600 mg twice daily), or another potent inhibitor of CYP2C8, and rosiglitazone (4 mg once daily) could increase the efficacy but also the risk of concentration-dependent adverse effects of rosiglitazone. Given the potential for dose-related adverse events with rosiglitazone, a decrease in the dose of rosiglitazone may be needed when gemfibrozil is introduced [1].

Rosiglitazone and Acarbose

Acarbose administered at therapeutic doses has a small, but clinically insignificant, effect on rosiglitazone pharmacokinetics. Rosiglitazone absorption was unaffected by acarbose. These observed changes in AUC(0-infinity) and t1/2 are not likely to be clinically relevant [2].

Rosiglitazone and Oral Contraceptives

The effect of rosiglitazone on the pharmacokinetics of ethinylestradiol and norethindrone was evaluated after repeat dosing of rosiglitazone with an oral contraceptive in a randomized, double-blind, placebo-controlled crossover study. Rosiglitazone had no significant effects on the pharmacokinetics of ethinylestradiol or norethindrone. Coadministration of rosiglitazone with contraceptive pills does not induce metabolism of these synthetic sex steroids and is not expected to impair the efficacy of contraceptive pills or hormone replacement therapy [3].

Rosiglitazone and Nifedipine

To examine the effects of repeat oral dosing of rosiglitazone on the pharmacokinetics of nifedipine, a prototype CYP3A4 substrate, a randomized, open-label, crossover study was performed. Rosiglitazone had no marked effect on nifedipine peak plasma concentration or time to peak concentration compared with nifedipine alone. Rosiglitazone coadministration produced a small decrease in the mean nifedipine half-life. Rosiglitazone, at the highest dose used in clinical studies, produced a small, clinically insignificant decrease in nifedipine exposure. The very small effect on nifedipine pharmacokinetics suggests that rosiglitazone is an extremely weak inducer of CYP3A4, a characteristic that distinguishes rosiglitazone from troglitazone [4].

Rosiglitazone and Digoxin

The potential for a drug-drug interaction with oral digoxin was investigated. Coadministration of digoxin with rosiglitazone had no significant effect on the safety or steady-state pharmacokinetics of digoxin [5].

Rosiglitazone and Ranitidine

The absolute bioavailability of rosiglitazone was 99%, and the oral and IV single-dose pharmacokinetics of rosiglitazone were unaltered by concurrent treatment with ranitidine [6].

Rosiglitazone and Sucralfate

No significant interactions between sucralfate and rosigliutazone have been observed [7].

Pharmacokinetics of Rosiglitazone in Patients with Renal Insufficiency

The pharmacokinetics of rosiglitazone was not markedly affected by mild, moderate, or severe renal insufficiency. Therefore, the starting dose of rosiglitazone does not need to be adjusted in patients with renal impairment [8].

HIGHLIGHTS

Rosiglitazone can be safely co-administred with the majority of the drugs used for the treatment of patients with metabolic syndrome. However, some potential interactions between rosiglitazone and gemfibrozil have been reported.

References

[1] Niemi M, Backman JT, Granfors M, Laitila J, Neuvonen M, Neuvonen PJ Gemfibrozil considerably increases the plasma concentrations of rosiglitazone. *Diabetologia*. 2003 Oct;46(10):1319-23.

[2] Miller AK, Inglis AM, Culkin KT, Jorkasky DK, Freed MI The effect of acarbose on the pharmacokinetics of rosiglitazone. *Eur J Clin Pharmacol.* 2001 May;57(2):105-9.

[3] Inglis AM, Miller AK, Culkin KT, Finnerty D, Patterson SD, Jorkasky DK, Freed MI. Lack of effect of rosiglitazone on the pharmacokinetics of oral contraceptives in healthy female volunteers. *J Clin Pharmacol.* 2001 Jun;41(6):683-90.
[4] Harris RZ, Inglis AM, Miller AK, Thompson KA, Finnerty D, Patterson S, Jorkasky DK, Freed MI. Rosiglitazone has no clinically significant effect on nifedipine pharmacokinetics. *J Clin Pharmacol.* 1999 Nov;39(11):1189-94.
[5] Di Cicco RA, Miller AK, Patterson S, Freed MI. Rosiglitazone does not affect the steady-state pharmacokinetics of digoxin. *J Clin Pharmacol.* 2000 Dec;40(12 Pt 2):1516-21.
[6] Miller AK, DiCicco RA, Freed MI The effect of ranitidine on the pharmacokinetics of rosiglitazone in healthy adult male volunteers. *Clin Ther.* 2002 Jul;24(7):1062-71.
[7] Rao MN, Mullangi R, Katneni K, Ravikanth B, Babu AP, Rani UP, Naidu MU, Srinivas NR, Rajagopalan R Lack of effect of sucralfate on the absorption and pharmacokinetics of rosiglitazone. *J Clin Pharmacol.* 2002 Jun;42(6):670-5.
[8] Chapelsky MC, Thompson-Culkin K, Miller AK, Sack M, Blum R, Freed MI Pharmacokinetics of rosiglitazone in patients with varying degrees of renal insufficiency. *J Clin Pharmacol.* 2003 Mar;43(3):252-9.

PIOGLITAZONE

Brief Compound Description

Pioglitazone [±)-5-[[4-[2-(5-ethyl-2-pyridinyl)ethoxy]phenyl]methyl]-2,4-] thiazolidinedione monohydrochloride. The molecule contains one asymmetric carbon, and the compound is synthesized and used as the racemic mixture. The two enantiomers of pioglitazone interconvert in vivo. No differences were found in the pharmacologic activity between the two enantiomers. The structural formula is as shown:

Drug Interactions

In humans, pioglitazone undergoes extensive metabolism, yielding primarily keto (M-III) and hydroxy (M-IV) derivatives of pioglitazone. The hepatic metabolism of pioglitazone is catalyzed mainly by CYP2C8 and CYP3A.23. Pioglitazone has been shown not to significantly affect major P450 activities using recombinant human P450 systems17 and in human liver microsomes [1].

Pioglitazone and Simvastatin

Pioglitazone does not alter the pharmacokinetics of the coadministered drugs simvastatin [2].

Pioglitazone and Atorvastatin

Clinical significant adverese events when rosiglitazone or pioglitazone and atorvastatin are administred together have been reported with controversial data. On the basis of adverse events reported to the US Food and Drug Administration, it was observed that atorvastatin-associated adverse event reports were 3.1 times more likely to list rosiglitazone or pioglitazone as a concomitant medication compared with simvastatin-associated adverse event reports [3].

Pioglitazone and Oral Contraceptive Pill

Pioglitazone does not alter the pharmacokinetics of ethinylestradiol, or norethindrone (CYP3A4 substrates) [4-5].

Pioglitazone and Sulphonylureas

No interactions between pioglitazone and glyburide, or glipizide (CYP2C9 substrates) have been recorded [4-5].

Pioglitazone and Warfarin

No interactions between pioglitazone and warfarin (CYP2C9 substrate) have been described [4-5].

References

[1] U.S. Package Circular: ACTOS®, July 1999.

[2] Liu L, Roadcap BA, Dilzer S, Lasseter KC, Rogers JD Interactions between simvastatin and troglitazone or pioglitazone in healthy subjects. *J Clin Pharmacol.* 2001 May;41(5):573-81

[3] Alsheikh-Ali AA, Karas RHAdverse events with concomitant use of simvastatin or atorvastatin and thiazolidinediones. *Am J Cardiol.* 2004 Jun 1;93(11):1417-8, A9.

[4] Carey R, Liu Y Pioglitazone does not markedly alter oral contraceptive or hormone replacement pharmacokinetics. *Diabetes* 2000; 49 (Suppl 1): A340-A341.

[5] Gillies P, Dunn C. Pioglitazone. *Drugs* 2000; 60: 333-343.

α-GLUCOSIDASE INHIBITORS

There are 3 α-glucosidase inhibitors: acarbose was released first, miglitol has just recently been marketed in the United States, and voglibose is not yet widely available. Although they can be used as monotherapy for type 2 diabetes mellitus, these antihyperglycemic drugs are frequently used in combination with the sulfonylureas or insulin.

Acarbose

Brief Compound Description

The chemical name of Acarbose O-4,6-Dideooxy-4-[[[1S-4R,5S,6S]]-4,5,6-triidroxy-3-(idroxymetyl)-2-cycloesen-1-yl]-amino]-a-D-glucopyranosyl (1, 4)-O-a-D-glucopyranosyl-

(1,4)-D-glucose. The molecular formula: C25H43NO18; the molecular weight is 645.63. The structural formula is the following:

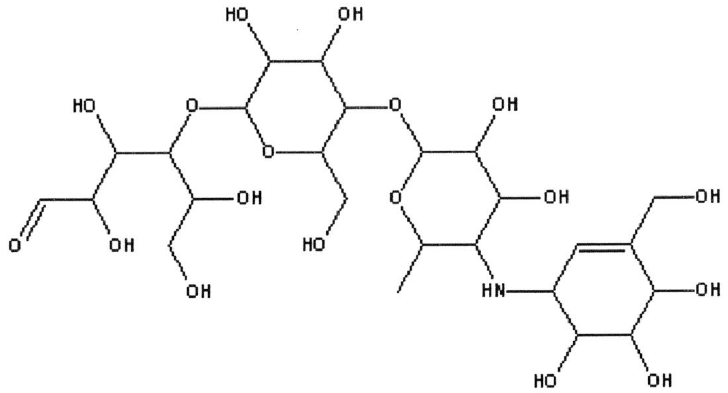

Miglitol

1,5-Dideoxy-1,5-[2-Hydroxyethyl)imino]-D-glucitol
The structural formula is the following:

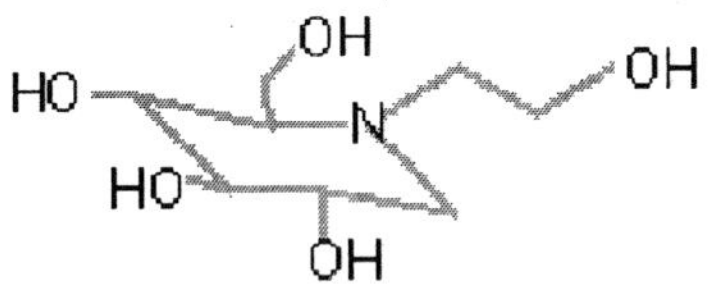

Mechanism of Action

These agents competitively and reversibly inhibit α-glucosidase, an intestinal brush border hydrolase enzyme. This leads to a postprandial decrease in carbohydrate absorption because complex dietary polysaccharides are not broken down into absorbable monosaccharides. As a result, there is a decrease in hyperinsulinism and in hepatic triglyceride synthesis. Lactose absorption is not affected because lactase is a -galactosidase. Acarbose is poorly absorbed; its mechanism of action is dependent on its local effects, as is its side effect profile.

Miglitol is rapidly and fully absorbed at low doses. Its antihyperglycemic mechanism of action is similar to that of acarbose; the implications of its systemic absorption are unknown. Hypothetically, because miglitol is cleared by the kidney, its use in patients with significant renal impairment may lead to As might be expected, the side effect profile of the α-glucosidase inhibitors is predominantly gastrointestinal because of their limited absorption.

Drug Interactions

There are no published reports of drug interactions overdose or severe toxicity with the α-glucosidase inhibitors. Possible drug interaction with the new anticholesterolemic drug ezetimibe will be evaluated.

INCRETINS

In this paragraph new and promising compounds for the treatment of type 2 diabetes, called "incretins" are briefly discussed. Obviously, very few drug-drug interactions have been reported.

EXENATIDE

Exenatide is the first in a new class of medicines known as incretin mimetics under investigation for the treatment of type 2 diabetes. Exenatide is an incretin mimetic with potential glucoregulatory activity in type 2 diabetes. The most frequent adverse events were generally mild to moderate nausea and vomiting.

Drug Interactions

Exenatide and acetaminophen Exenatide treatment concurrent with or preceding acetaminophen ingestion slowed acetaminophen absorption but had minimal effect on the extent of absorption [1].

GLUCAGON-LIKE PEPTIDE-1 (GLP-1)

Glucagon-like peptide-1 (GLP-1) is a proglucagon-derived peptide secreted from gut endocrine cells in response to nutrient ingestion. The multifaceted actions of GLP-1 include the following: (1) the stimulation of insulin secretion and of its gene expression, (2) the inhibition of glucagon secretion, (3) the inhibition of food intake, (4) the proliferation and differentiation of beta cells, and (5) the protection of beta-cells from apoptosis. The therapeutic utility of the native GLP-1 molecule is limited by its rapid enzymatic degradation by a serine protease termed dipeptidyl peptidase-IV (DPP-IV). [1-2]

Main References

[1] Blase E, Taylor K, Gao HY, Wintle M, Fineman M. Pharmacokinetics of an oral drug (acetaminophen) administered at various times in relation to subcutaneous injection of exenatide (exendin-4) in healthy subjects. *J Clin Pharmacol.* 2005 May;45(5):570-7.

[2] Hui H, Zhao X, Perfetti R Structure and function studies of glucagon-like peptide-1 (GLP-1): the designing of a novel pharmacological agent for the treatment of diabetes. *Diabetes Metab Res Rev.* 2005 Apr 26.

[3] Vilsboll T, Holst JJ: Incretins, insulin secretion and type 2 diabetes mellitus. *Diabetologia* 47:357 –366,2004.

Chapter 4

LIPID-LOWERING AGENTS

HMG-COA REDUCTASE INHIBITORS (STATINS)

The 3-hydroxy-3-methylglutaryl coenzyme A (HMG-CoA) reductase inhibitors, widely called statins: atorvastatin, fluvastatin, pravastatin, lovastatin, and simvastatin, can achieve relatively large reductions in plasma cholesterol levels and are a well-established class of drugs for the treatment of hypercholesterolemia. Since statins are prescribed on a long-term basis, possible interactions with other drugs deserve attention as many patients will typically receive multiple-drug treatment for concomitant conditions during the course of statin therapy. At the pharmacodynamic level, statins are not prone to interference with other drugs. At the pharmacokinetic level, however, interactions can affect the processes by which statins are absorbed, distributed, metabolized, and excreted.

Brief Compounds Description

Simvastatin, an inactive lactone, is hydrolyzed to the corresponding (beta)-hydroxyacid form, which is an inhibitor of HMG-CoA reductase. Simvastatin is butanoic acid, 2,2-dimethyl,1,2,3,7,8,8a-hexahydro-3,7- dimethyl-8-[2-(tetrahydro-4-hydroxy-6-oxo-2 *H* -pyran-2-yl)-ethyl]-1-naphthalenyl ester, [1 *S* - [1(alpha),3(alpha),7(beta),8(beta)(2 *S* *,4 *S* *),-8a(beta]]. The empirical formula of simvastatin is $C_{25}H_{38}O_5$ and its molecular weight is 418.57.

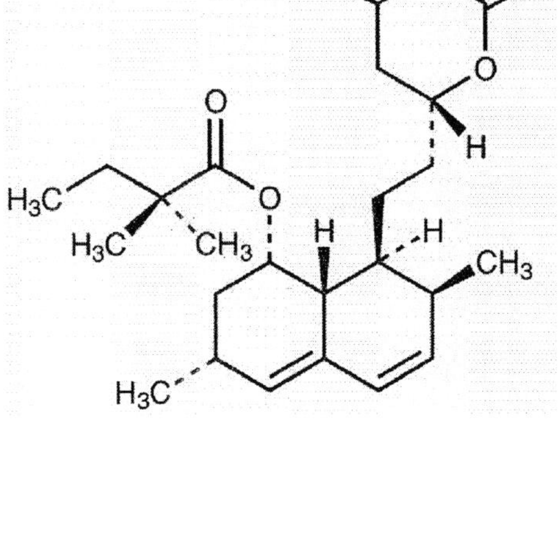

Pravastatin sodium is designated chemically as 1-Naphthalene-heptanoic acid, 1,2,6,7,8,8a-hexahydro-(beta),(delta),6-trihydroxy-2-methyl-8-(2-methyl-1-oxobutoxy)-, monosodium salt, [1S-[1(alpha)((beta)S*,(delta)S*),2(alpha),6(alpha),8(beta)(R*),8a(alpha]] -. Structural formula

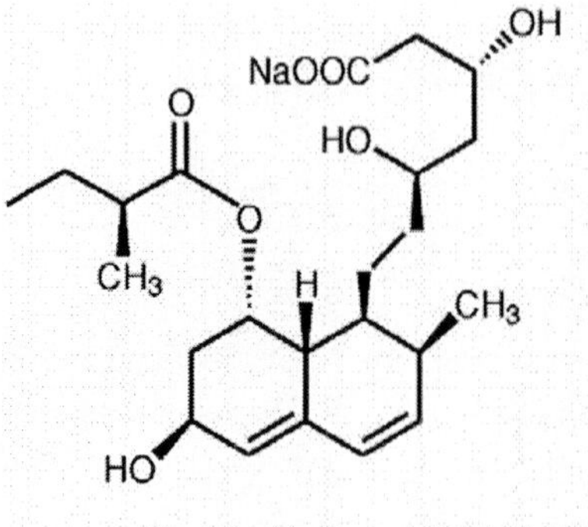

$C_{23}H_{35}NaO_7$ MW 446.52

Fluvastatin sodium is [*R**, *S* *-(*E*]-(±)-7-[3-(4-fluorophenyl)-1-(1-methylethyl)-1 *H* -indol-2-yl]-3,5-dihydroxy-6-heptenoic acid, monosodium salt. The empirical formula of fluvastatin sodium is $C_{24}H_{25}FNO_4 \cdot Na$, its molecular weight is 433.46 and its structural formula is

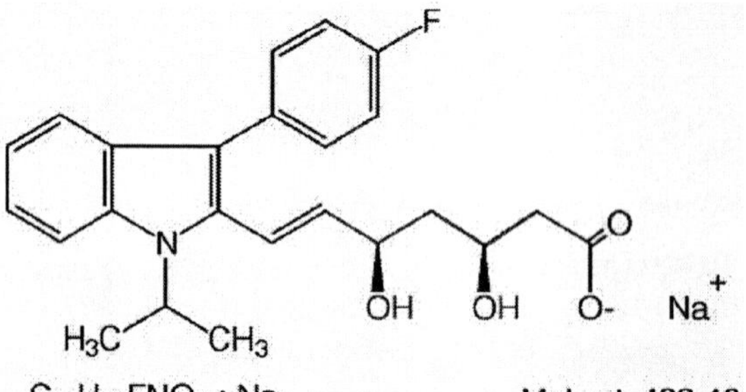

$C_{24}H_{25}FNO_4 \cdot Na$ Mol. wt. 433.46

Rosuvastatin calcium is bis[E)-7-[4-(4-fluorophenyl)-6-isopropyl-2-[methyl (methylsulfonyl)amino] pyrimidin-5-yl](3R,5S)-3,5-dihydroxyhept-6-enoic acid] calcium salt. The empirical formula for rosuvastatin calcium is $(C_{22}H_{27}FN_3O_6S)_2Ca$. Its molecular weight is 1001.14. Its structural formula is:

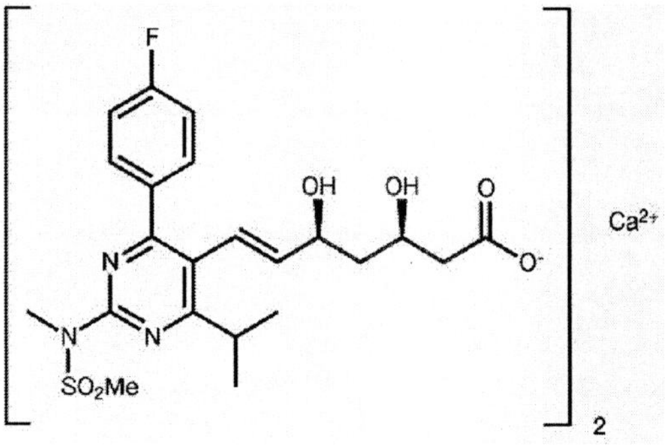

Atorvastatin calcium is [R-(R*, R*]-2-(4-fluorophenyl)-(beta), (delta)-dihydroxy-5-(1-methylethyl)-3-phenyl-4-[phenylamino)carbonyl]-1H-pyrrole-1-heptanoic acid, calcium salt (2:1) trihydrate. The empirical formula of atorvastatin calcium is $(C_{33}H_{34}FN_2O_5)_2Ca \cdot 3H_2O$ and its molecular weight is 1209.42. Its structural formula is:

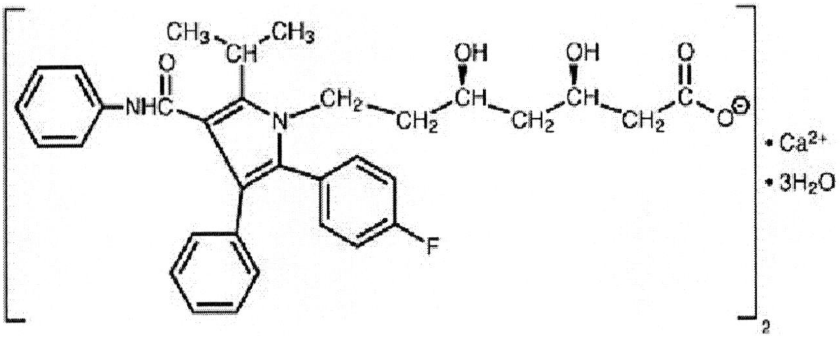

Lovastatin is [1 *S* -[1(alpha)(*R*),3(alpha),7(beta),8(beta)(2 *S*, 4 *S*),8a(beta]]-1,2,3,7,8,8a-hexahydro-3,7-dimethyl-8-[2-(tetrahydro-4-hydroxy-6-oxo-2 *H* -pyran-2-yl)ethyl]-1-naphthalenyl 2-methylbutanoate. The empirical formula of lovastatin is $C_{24}H_{36}O_5$ and its molecular weight is 404.55. Its structural formula is:

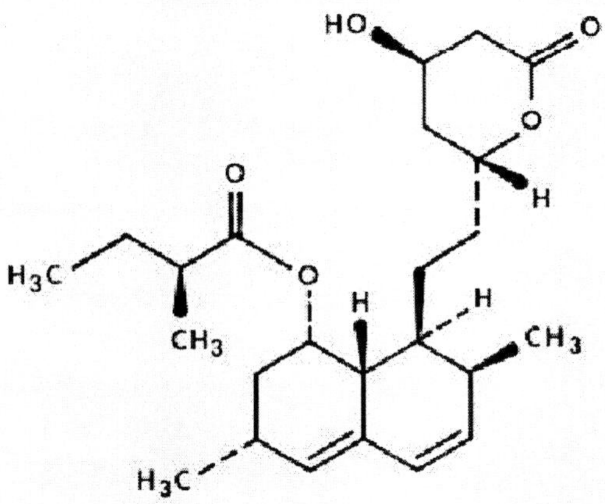

General Drug Interaction

Many drug–drug interactions have been demonstrated in clinical experience with statins and in many respects these interactions are qualitatively and quantitatively comparable for all agents of this class. Some of these interactions are indeed of minor clinical consequence because they neither compromise cholesterol-lowering activity nor increase toxicity. Due to differences in statin physicochemical and pharmacokinetic properties, however, some important differences in their interaction potential have been reported (table 1). Of particular note are interactions with other lipid-lowering agents used for treatment of patients with metabolic syndrome, such as fibrates and niacin (nicotinic acid), warfarin, [1].

Drug Interactions With Statins: Focus on Pharmacokinetic Differences

Table 1. Drugs That May Increase Risk of Myopathy and Rhabdomyolysis When Used Concomitantly With Statins

Statin
Potentially Interacting Drugs
Simvastatin
Mibefradil
Fibrates
Cyclosporine
Warfarin
Digoxin
Niacin
Atorvastatin
Mibefradil
Fibrates
Warfarin
Cyclosporine
Digoxin
Pravastatin
Fibrates
Warfarin
Cyclosporine
Digoxin
Mibefradil
Niacin
Lovastatin
Cyclosporine Warfarin
Niacin
Fibrates
Digoxin
Mibefradil
Fluvastatin
Fibrates
Warfarin
Digoxin
Mibefradil
Sildenafil
Rosuvastatin
Warfarin
Fibrates

Modified from Omar MA, Wilson JP. Ann Pharmacother. 2002;36:288–295.

To understand the molecular bases of statin-drug interactions, it is important to mention that statins are very selective inhibitors of HMG-CoA reductase and usually do not show any relevant affinity toward other enzymes or receptor systems. This suggests that, at the pharmacodynamic level statins are not prone to interfere with other drugs. However, at the pharmacokinetic level, the available statins have important differences, including half-life, systemic exposure, maximum plasma concentration (Cmax), bioavailability, protein binding, lipophilicity, metabolism, presence of active metabolites, and excretion routes. With the exception of pravastatin, which is transformed enzymatically in the liver cytosol, all statins undergo extensive microsomal metabolism by the cytochrome P450 (CYP) isoenzyme systems. Pharmacokinetic interactions resulting in myositis and rhabdomyolysis have been reported after concurrent use of statins and several different classes of drugs (table 1).

The CYP3A4 isoenzyme is responsible for the metabolism of lovastatin, simvastatin, and atorvastatin. Fluvastatin (metabolized by CYP 2C9) and pravastatin (eliminated by other metabolic routes) are less subject to this interaction. Rosuvastatin is not extensively metabolized, but has some interaction with the CYP2C9 enzyme. These differences can affect the potential for drug interactions with statins, which can result in markedly increased or decreased plasma concentrations of some drugs within this class. Since statins have different pharmacological properties, some statins may be more or less likely than others to cause drug interactions. Nevertheless, the incidence of both myopathy and rhabdomyolysis with statins is quite low, despite the common coprescription of these agents with competing substrates or inhibitors of their metabolism.

Metabolic syndrome drugs showing clinically significant interactions with statins or with a potential, but lower risk are summarized in Table 2.

Table 2. Drugs showing not or only potential interactions with Statins in metabolic syndrome

NO	Potential
Ezetimibe	Bezafibrate
	Fenofibrate
Propranolol	
Thiazide diuretics	
ACE inhibitors	
Sartans	
Ximelagatran	

Drug Interactions

Statins and Fibric Acid Derivatives (Fibrates)

The interaction of statins with fibrates deserves particular attention because myopathy can occur with either drug alone, and the effects may be additive [2]. Although all fibrates have been associated with cases of CK elevations and myopathy in combination with statins, the risk for the development of myopathy may be greater for gemfibrozil compared with bezafibrate or fenofibrate. The concomitant use of gemfibrozil and atorvastatin, lovastatin, pravastatin, or simvastatin has been associated with case reports of rhabdomyolysis.

Gemfibrozil was shown to increase plasma concentrations of active simvastatin and lovastatin acid forms but minimally the lactone forms, whereas bezafibrate demonstrated no significant effect on the pharmacokinetics of lovastatin and simvastatin [3-4]. Recently, it was shown that gemfibrozil can modulate the pharmacokinetics of statins more via inhibition of statin hydroxy acid glucuronidation than via inhibition of CYP3A4-mediated oxidation. Glucuronidation is a previously unrecognized, but common, metabolic pathway for the conversion of active open acid forms of several statins (including atorvastatin and rosuvastatin) to their lactone form. The lactone form, in turn, plays a critical role in the subsequent statin metabolism catalyzed by CYP3A4. Additionally, a potential difference between gemfibrozil and fenofibrate in their ability to alter the pharmacokinetics of statins has been shown in human hepatocytes where fenofibrate was much less effective than gemfibrozil in affecting simvastatin metabolism. Finally, the interaction between gemfibrozil and pravastatin could occur at the transport protein level.

The effect of gemfibrozil on rosuvastatin pharmacokinetics was assessed in healthy volunteers. Rosuvastatin has been shown to be a substrate for the human hepatic uptake transporter organic anion transporter 2 (OATP2). Inhibition of this transporter could increase plasma concentrations of rosuvastatin. The effect of gemfibrozil on rosuvastatin uptake by cells expressing OATP2 was also examined. Gemfibrozil increased rosuvastatin plasma concentrations approximately 2-fold, which is similar to the effect of gemfibrozil on pravastatin, simvastatin acid, and lovastatin acid plasma concentrations and substantially less than the effect observed for cerivastatin. Gemfibrozil inhibition of OATP2-mediated rosuvastatin hepatic uptake may contribute to the mechanism of the drug-drug interaction [5].

Nevertheless, a body of evidences showed that no clinically significant drug interactions between statins and fibrates occur. In fact, no cases of myopathy have been described in patients receiving both lovastatin and bezafibrate [6]. Concomitant administration of fenofibrate and pravastatin did not affect the pharmacokinetics of either fenofibric acid or pravastatin [7] and no clinically significant pharmacokinetic drug interaction between fenofibrate and simvastatin was concluded in humans [8].

Statins and Calcium Channel Blockers

Metabolic syndrome patients may require the co-prescription of calcium antagonists such as diltiazem or verapamil that are weak inhibitors of CYP 3A4. The co-administration of diltiazem with lovastatin or simvastatin caused a fourfold increase in plasma concentrations of both statins [9]. Diltiazem greatly increased the plasma concentration of lovastatin, but the magnitude of this effect was much greater than that predicted by the systemic serum concentration, suggesting that this interaction is a first-pass rather than a systemic event [10]. This interaction is most probably due to a first-pass effect, since the intravenous administration of diltiazem did not significantly affect the pharmacokinetic bioavailability of lovastatin. Intravenous diltiazem did not significantly affect the oral AUC, Cmax, t, or tmax of lovastatin. These data suggest that the interaction of lovastatin with diltiazem does not occur systemically and is primarily a first-pass effect. Thus, drug interactions with diltiazem may become evident when a patient is moved from intravenous to oral dosing [11-12]. In addition, two cases of rhabdomyolysis have been reported with diltiazem and simvastatin [13-14]. Drug interactions between calcium antagonist mibefradil and simvastatin or lovastatin have been reported. Mibefradil is metabolized by two hepatic pathways: hydrolysis of the ester bond in the side chain and oxidation by CYP 3A4. Metabolism by the oxidative pathway is inhibited after long-term administration of mibefradil, thus leading to possible interactions with other agents metabolized through the same pathway. Indeed, 19 cases of simvastatin-associated rhabdomyolysis and one case with lovastatin have been reported in patients receiving mibefradil. Plasma concentrations of simvastatin and its active metabolite (-hydroxy-simvastatin) were increased as a result of the inhibition of their metabolism by mibefradil. Mibefradil and its metabolite inhibit not only CYP 3A4 but also CYP 1A2 and CYP 2D6. Therefore, increased plasma concentrations of drugs metabolized by these isoenzymes could be expected when co-administered with mibefradil. The active metabolites

of simvastatin are biotransformed by CYP 2D6, which could have potentiated the interaction with mibefradil [15].
By the contrast some reports found no interactions between ca-antagonists and statins. Approximately, one-third of patients randomized to simvastatin were receiving concomitant medication with a calcium channel blocker, and the data provide no evidence that concomitant use of calcium channel blockers such as diltiazem and verapamil increases the risk of simvastatin-associated myopathy. Also post-marketing analysis of the clinical use of statins concomitantly with calcium antagonists did not give any signal of a clinically significant interactive effect for either simvastatin or pravastatin [16].

Statins and Glitazones

Cytochrome P450 inducers might reduce statin plasma levels. This seems to be the case with troglitazone, an antidiabetic agent that otherwise has been withdrawn from the market [17].

Statins and Anticouagulants

Interaction can occur between statins and coumarin anticoagulants. Although the administration of lovastatin to patients receiving warfarin had no effect on prothrombin time, bleeding and/or increased anticoagulant effects have been reported in several patients taking anticoagulants concomitantly with lovastatin. Simvastatin normally causes only a small, clinically irrelevant increase of the anticoagulant effects of warfarin [18]. Nevertheless, a more marked anticoagulant effect and bruising have been seen in one patient and a case of rhabdomyolysis and acute renal failure associated with concomitant use of simvastatin and warfarin has been described. Warfarin, which is known to be metabolized, at least in part, by the same CYP3 A4 isoform of the hepatic microsomal P450 system, may increase simvastatin serum levels. There are no studies directly examining the effect of warfarin on simvastatin serum levels, but there is evidence for an interaction between the two drugs as manifest by a prolongation of the INR when simvastatin or lovastatin is administered upon a stable dose of warfarin [19].

One case report describes an interaction between simvastatin and the anticoagulant acenocoumarol, which resulted in an elevated INR. Pravastatin does not appear to interact with warfarin but has caused an increased INR when combined with the anticoagulant fluindione. Clinicians should monitor the INR closely after starting statin therapy in any patient receiving anticoagulation therapy [20].

Conflicting data have been reported on the effect of statins on clopidogrel-inhibited platelet aggregation in patients undergoing coronary stenting; at the moment, there are no clear reasons to exclude the coadministration of these two classes of drugs in patients who are at high risk for coronary events. Statins primarily metabolized by cytochrome P450 3A4 (CYP3A4) reportedly reduce clopidogrel's metabolism to active metabolite, thus attenuating its inhibition of platelet aggregation ex vivo. Although ex vivo testing has suggested a potential negative interaction when coadministering a CYP3A4-metabolized statin with clopidogrel, this was not clinically observed statistically in a post hoc analysis of a placebo-controlled study [21]. No pharmacokinetic or pharmacodynamic interaction between atorvastatin and ximelagatran was observed [22].

Statin and Niacin Potential interaction between nicotinic acid (niacin) and statin has been reported. Nevertheless, clinical trials in which patients have received niacin in combination with fluvastatin, pravastatin, or simvastatin have also not reported myopathy. Myopathy has been reported in 2% of patients receiving lovastatin in combination with niacin [23]. The mechanism behind this interaction is not completely elucidated. However, plasma concentrations of the active metabolites of lovastatin were not elevated in patients receiving niacin. It therefore remains unclear as to why niacin should precipitate myopathy in lovastatin-treated patients. An incidence of myopathy of 0.15% for lovastatin monotherapy, increasing to 2, 5, and 28%, respectively, in patients receiving concomitant niacin, cyclosporine A plus niacin, and cyclosporine A plus gemfibrozil [24] By the contrast no interactions have been documented when niacin was administered with simvastatin, fluvastatin, or pravastatin.

Statins and Digoxin

Digoxin is a P-glycoprotein substrate/inhibitor, a class of active drug transporters, including the P-glycoproteins, is known to affect the disposition and bioavailability of many drugs, including CYP3A4 substrates. Transport proteins are, at least in part, responsible for the low and variable oral bioavailability of atorvastatin, lovastatin, simvastatin, and pravastatin Indeed, interactions with other drugs at the P-glycoprotein level could potentially be responsible for the rhabdomyolysis observed after statin-digoxin combination therapy. Rosuvastatin, but not fluvastatin, has been shown to be recognized by these transporters. Rosuvastatin is metabolized slowly and to a limited extent in the liver involving the CYP isoenzymes 2C9 and 2C19. Thus, it is unlikely that rosuvastatin will participate in metabolic-based drug interactions. Only one clinical relevant interaction has been observed between simvastatin or atorvastatin and digoxin, which caused a slight elevation in plasma digoxin concentrations leading to an increased cardiac activity.

Statins and Propranolol, and Thiazide Diuretics

No clinically important interactions have been observed between statins and other drugs used in cardiovascular diseases, such as propranolol, and thiazide diuretics.

Statins and Angiotensin-converting-enzyme Inhibitors and Sartans

Irbesartan had no significant effect on the single-dose pharmacokinetics of total simvastatin acid [25].

Fluvastatin did not significantly change the steady-state AUC0-24 or half-life of losartan. Losartan apparent oral clearance was not affected by fluvastatin [26].

Simvastatin and Ezetimibe

No cases of rhabdomyolysis when ezetimibe and simvastatin were co-administred [27].

Statins and Dialysis

If subtle differences may exist in the metabolic processing of atorvastatin in haemodialysis patients, active drug did not accumulate nor did it show enhanced elimination, and levels were comparable to those measured in healthy volunteers. Therefore there is no need to adapt atorvastatin dosage in this particular patient population [28]

Alzheimer's Disease and Statins

Cognitive impairment and dementia as potential adverse effects associated with statin therapy have been reported [29]

HIGHLIGHTS

Statins can potentially interact with some of the drugs used for the treatment of patients with metabolic syndrome, as well as fibrates, calcium channels antagonists, anticoagulants, niacin. However, among statins, fluvastatin, pravastatin and rosuvastatin have been reported to be less subject to CYP3A4 interactions. Other drugs, such as ezetimibe, thiazide diuretics, ACE-inhibitors, sartans and beta-blockers have been not found to interact with statins. Finally, among fibrates, fenofibrate seems to be more safely co-administred with statins.

REFERENCES

[1] Paoletti R, Corsini A, Bellosta S Pharmacological interactions of statins. *Atheroscler Suppl.* 2002 May;3(1):35-40.

[2] P. Pauciullo, C. Borgnino, R. Paoletti, M. Mariani and M. Mancini, Efficacy and safety of a combination of fluvastatin and bezafibrate in patients with mixed hyperlipidaemia FACT study. *Atherosclerosis* 2000; 150: 429–436.

[3] Schneck DW, Birmingham BK, Zalikowski JA, Mitchell PD, Wang Y, Martin PD, Lasseter KC, Brown CD, Windass AS, Raza A. The effect of gemfibrozil on the pharmacokinetics of rosuvastatin. *Clin Pharmacol Ther.* 2004 May;75(5):455-63.

[4] P. Pauciullo, C. Borgnino, R. Paoletti, M. Mariani and M. Mancini, Efficacy and safety of a combination of fluvastatin and bezafibrate in patients with mixed hyperlipidaemia FACT study. *Atherosclerosis* 2000; 150: 429–436.

[5] Pan WJ, Gustavson LE, Achari R, Rieser MJ, Ye X, Gutterman C, Wallin BALack of a clinically significant pharmacokinetic interaction between fenofibrate and pravastatin in healthy volunteers. *J Clin Pharmacol.* 2000 Mar;40(3):316-23.

[6] Bergman AJ, Murphy G, Burke J, Zhao JJ, Valesky R, Liu L, Lasseter KC, He W, Prueksaritanont T, Qiu Y, Hartford A, Vega JM, Paolini JFSimvastatin does not have a clinically significant pharmacokinetic interaction with fenofibrate in humans. *J Clin Pharmacol.* 2004 Sep;44(9):1054-62.

[7] R.A. Boyd, R.H. Stern, B.H. Stewart, X. Wu, E.L. Reyner, E.A. Zegarac, E.J. Randinitis and L. Whitfield, Atorvastatin coadministration may increase digoxin concentrations by inhibition of intestinal P-glycoprotein-mediated secretion. *J. Clin. Pharmacol.* 40 (2000), pp. 91–98.

[8] Lins RL, Matthys KE, Verpooten GA, Peeters PC, Dratwa M, Stolear JC, Lameire NHPharmacokinetics of atorvastatin and its metabolites after single and multiple dosing in hypercholesterolaemic haemodialysis patients. *Nephrol Dial Transplant.* 2003 May;18(5):967-76.

[9] N.E. Azie, D.C. Brater, P.A. Becker, D.R. Jones and S.D. Hall. The interaction of diltiazem with lovastatin and pravastatin. *Clin. Pharmacol. Ther.* 64 (1998), pp. 369–377.

[10] O. Mousa, D.C. Brater, K.J. Sunblad, S.D. Hall. The interaction of diltiazem with simvastatin. *Clin. Pharmacol. Ther.* 2000; 67: 267–274.

[11] A.L. Masica, N.E. Azie, D.C. Brater, S.D. Hall, D.R. Jones. Intravenous diltiazem and CYP 3A-mediated metabolism. *Br. J. Clin. Pharmacol.* 2000; 50: 273–276.

[12] K.R. Yeo, W.W. Yeo, E.J. Wallis. L.E. Ramsay, Enhanced cholesterol reduction by simvastatin in diltiazem-treated patients. *Br. J. Clin. Pharmacol.* 199; 48:: 610–615

[13] N. Kanathur, M.G. Mathai, R.P. Byrd, Jr., C.L. Fields, T.M. Roy, Simvastatin–diltiazem drug interaction resulting in rhabdomyolysis and hepatitis. *Tenn. Med.* 2001; 94: 339–341.

[14] R. Peces, A. Pobes, Rhabdomyolysis associated with concurrent use of simvastatin and diltiazem. *Nephron* 2001; 89: 117–118.

[15] D. Schmassmann-Suhijar, R. Bullingham, R. Gasser, J. Schmutz, W.E. Haefeli, Rhabdomyolysis due to interaction of simvastatin with mibefradil. *Lancet* 1998; 351:1929–1930.

[16] P.J.K. Gruer, J.M. Vega, M.F. Mercuri, M.R. Dobrinska, J.A. Tobert, Concomitant use of cytochrome P450 3A4 inhibitors and simvastatin. *Am. J. Cardiol.* 1999; 84: 811–815.

[17] J.C. Lin, M.K. Ito, A drug interaction between troglitazone and simvastatin. *Diabetes Care* 1999; 22:. 2104–2105.

[18] Stern R, Abel R, Gibson GL, Besserer J.Atorvastatin does not alter the anticoagulant activity of warfarin. *J Clin Pharmacol.* 1997 Nov;37(11):1062-4.

[19] Mogyorosi, B. Bradley, A. Showalter, M.L. Schubert, Rhabdomyolysis and acute renal failure due to combination therapy with simvastatin and warfarin. *J. Intern. Med.* 1999; 246: 599–602.

[20] Andrus MR Oral anticoagulant drug interactions with statins: case report of fluvastatin and review of the literature. *Pharmacotherapy.* 2004 Feb;24(2):285-90.

[21] Saw J, Topol EJ.Lack of adverse clopidogrel-atorvastatin clinical interaction from secondary analysis of a randomized, placebo-controlled clopidogrel trial. *Circulation.* 2003 Aug 26;108(8):921-4.

[22] Sarich TC, Schutzer KM, Dorani H, Wall U, Kalies I, Ohlsson L, Eriksson UG No pharmacokinetic or pharmacodynamic interaction between atorvastatin and the oral direct thrombin inhibitor ximelagatran. *J Clin Pharmacol.* 2004 Aug;44(8):928-34.

[23] J. Shepherd Fibrates and statins in the treatment of hyperlipidaemia: an appraisal of their efficacy and safety. *Eur. Heart J.* 1995; 16: 5–13.

[24] J.T. Backman, C. Kyrklund, K.T. Kivisto, J.S. Wang, P.J. Neuvonen, Plasma concentrations of active simvastatin acid are increased by gemfibrozil. *Clin. Pharmacol. Ther.* 2000; 68: 122–129.

[25] Marino MR, Vachharajani NN, Hadjilambris OW. Irbesartan does not affect the pharmacokinetics of simvastatin in healthy subjects. *J Clin Pharmacol.* 2000 Aug;40(8):875-9.

[26] Meadowcroft AM, Williamson KM, Patterson JH, Hinderliter AL, Pieper JA. The effects of fluvastatin, a CYP2C9 inhibitor, on losartan pharmacokinetics in healthy volunteers. *J Clin Pharmacol.* 1999 Apr;39(4):418-24.

[27] Ballantyne CM, Blazing MA, King TR, Brady WE, Palmisano JEfficacy and safety of ezetimibe co-administered with simvastatin compared with atorvastatin in adults with hypercholesterolemia. *Am J Cardiol.* 2004 Jun 15;93(12):1487-94.

[28] Martin PD, Warwick MJ, Dane AL, Hill SJ, Giles PB, Phillips PJ, Lenz E. Metabolism, excretion, and pharmacokinetics of rosuvastatin in healthy adult male volunteers. *Clin Ther.* 2003 Nov;25(11):2822-35.
[29] King DS, Wilburn AJ, Wofford MR, Harrell TK, Lindley BJ, Jones DW.Cognitive impairment associated with atorvastatin and simvastatin. *Pharmacotherapy.* 2003 Dec;23(12):1663-7.

FIBRATES

Main Mechanisms of Action

Fibrates are lipid regulating agents which decrease serum triglycerides and very low density lipoprotein (VLDL) cholesterol, and increases high density lipoprotein (HDL) cholesterol. The mechanism of action of fibrates has not been definitely established. In man, fibrates have been shown to inhibit peripheral lipolysis and to decrease the hepatic extraction of free fatty acids, thus reducing hepatic triglyceride production. Fibrates inhibit synthesis and increases clearance of VLDL carrier apolipoprotein B, leading to a decrease in VLDL production. Animal studies suggest that fibrates may, in addition to elevating HDL-cholesterol, reduce incorporation of long-chain fatty acids into newly formed triglycerides, accelerate turnover and removal of cholesterol from the liver, and increase excretion of cholesterol in the feces.

The effects of fibrates, observed in clinical practice, have been explained in vivo in transgenic mice and in vitro in human hepatocyte cultures by the activation of peroxisome proliferator activated receptor (alpha) (PPAR(alpha)). Through this mechanism, fibrates increases lipolysis and elimination of triglyceride-rich particles from plasma by activating lipoprotein lipase and reducing production of apoproteins C-III (an inhibitor of lipoprotein lipase activity). The resulting fall in triglycerides produces an alteration in the size and composition of LDL from small, dense particles (which are thought to be atherogenic due to their susceptibility to oxidation), to large buoyant particles. These larger particles have a greater affinity for cholesterol receptors and are catabolized rapidly. Activation of PPARa also induces an increase in the synthesis of apoproteins A-I, A-II and HDL-cholesterol.

General Drug Interactions

In vitro studies using human liver microsomes indicate that fenofibrate and fenofibric acid are not inhibitors of cytochrome (CYP) P450 isoforms CYP3A4, CYP2D6, CYP2E1, or CYP1A2. They are weak inhibitors of CYP2C19 and CYP2A6, and mild-to-moderate inhibitors of CYP2C9 at therapeutic concentrations.

The combined use of fibric acid derivatives and HMG-CoA reductase inhibitors has been associated, in the absences of a marked pharmacokinetic interaction, in numerous case reports, with rhabdomyolysis, markedly elevated creatine kinase (CK) levels and myoglobinuria, leading in a high proportion of cases to acute renal failure.

Potentiation of coumarin-type anti-coagulants has been observed with prolongation of the prothrombin time/INR.

GEMFIBROZIL

Brief Compound Description

The chemical name is 5-(2,5-dimethylphenoxy)-2,2-dimethylpentanoic acid, the empirical formula is C15H22O3 and the molecular weight is 250.35.

Gemfibrozil has the following structural formula:

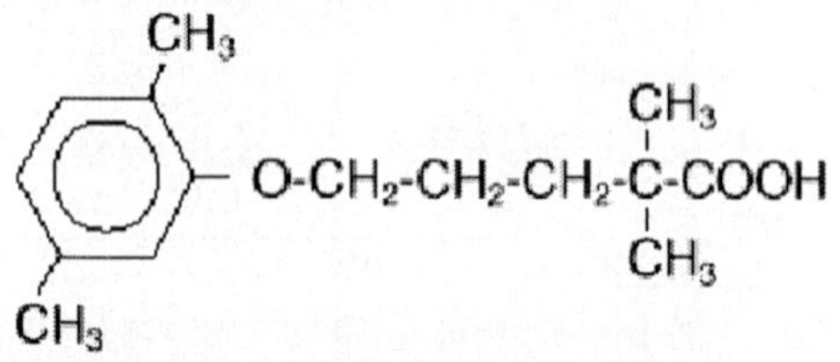

CH_3 CH_3 $O\text{-}CH_2\text{-}CH_2\text{-}CH_2\text{-}C\text{-}COOH$ CH_3 CH_3

Gemfibrozil is well absorbed from the gastrointestinal tract after oral administration. Peak plasma levels occur in 1 to 2 hours with a plasma half-life of 1.5 hours following multiple doses.

Drug Interactions

Main of the possible drug-drug interactions between Gemfibrozil and other components used in patients with metabolic syndrome are summarized in Table 1. The mechanisms and some of these potential interactions are discussed in detail below.

Table 1. Potential drug-drug interactions with Gemfibrozil in metabolic syndrome

YES	Mechanism and effect	NO
Simvastatin Lovastatin	⇑ increased concentration of statins, **myopathy**	Ezetimibe
Glimepiride Repaglinide	⇒ prolonged blood glucose-lowering effect	
Warfarin	⇒ prolongation of the prothrombin time/INR	

The in vitro inhibitory effects of gemfibrozil on cytochrome P450 (CYP) 1A2, CYP2A6, CYP2C9, CYP2C19, CYP2D6, CYP2E1, and CYP3A4 activities has been examined using pooled human liver microsomes. Gemfibrozil strongly and competitively inhibited CYP2C9 activity. In addition, gemfibrozil exhibited somewhat smaller inhibitory effects on CYP2C19 and CYP1A2 activities. Gemfibrozil inhibits the activity of CYP2C9 at clinically relevant concentrations, and this is the likely mechanism by which gemfibrozil interacts with CYP2C9 substrate drugs, such as warfarin and glyburide. Gemfibrozil may also impair clearance of CYP2C19 and CYP1A2 substrates, but inhibition of other CYP isoforms is unlikely [1].

Gemfibrozil and Statins

The risk of myopathy and rhabdomyolysis is increased with combined gemfibrozil and HMG-CoA reductase inhibitor therapy [2-5].

Preclinical studies have demonstrated that gemfibrozil-mediated elevations of simvastatin AUC after oral simvastatin administration to humans are not due to inhibitory effects of gemfibrozil on CYP3A-mediated metabolism of simvastatin, but are due, at least in part, to the inhibitory activity of gemfibrozil on competitive inhibitor of UDP-glucuronosyltransferase (UGT) isoforms UGT1A1- and/or UGT1A3-mediated glucuronidation of simvastatin. Some data suggest that gemfibrozil has the potential to modulate the pharmacokinetics of other statins, by inhibition of statin hydroxy acid glucuronidation. Moreover, various statins exhibit differential susceptibility to the inhibitory effects of gemfibrozil on their metabolic clearance via glucuronidation and/or non-CYP3A4-mediated oxidative pathways [6].

The in vitro rhCYP2C8 inhibitory potency observed for gemfibrozil is relatively weak, but gemfibrozil glucuronide has recently been shown to be a significantly more potent inhibitor of human CYP2C8 activity. Circulating concentrations of gemfibrozil glucuronide have been reported to be greater than the IC50 for CYP2C8, and therefore this metabolite could have a greater contribution to in vivo drug interactions than the parent drug [7].

The inhibitory effects of gemfibrozil and its metabolites, M3 and gemfibrozil 1-O-beta-glucuronide, on the uptake of cerivastatin by human organic anion transporting polypeptide 2 (OATP2)-expressing cells and its metabolism in cytochrome P450 expression systems has been studied [8].

Some differences between fibrates in pharmacokinetic interactions with statins have been suggested [9]. Gemfibrozil was not only found to moderately interact with the CYP3A4 pathway but was also found to be a strong inhibitor of the glucuronidation-mediated lactonization of several statins. In contrast, fenofibrate showed a minimal effect on all metabolic pathways, including the statin glucuronidation [10]. Gemfibrozil markedly increases plasma concentrations of lovastatin acid, but bezafibrate does not. The increased risk of myopathy observed during concomitant treatment with statins and fibrates may be partially of a pharmacokinetic origin. The risk of developing myopathy during concomitant therapy with lovastatin and a fibrate may be smaller with bezafibrate than with gemfibrozil [11].

Gemfibrozil and Ezetimibe

The coadministration of ezetimibe and gemfibrozil in patients is unlikely to cause a clinically significant drug interaction. In fact, ezetimibe did not alter the bioavailability of gemfibrozil. Conversely, gemfibrozil significantly increased the plasma concentrations of ezetimibe and total ezetimibe. Exposure to ezetimibe and total ezetimibe was increased approximately 1.4-fold and 1.7-fold, respectively, however, this increase was not considered to be clinically relevant [12].

Gemfibrozil and Repaglinide

Gemfibrozil considerably enhanced and prolonged the blood glucose-lowering effect of repaglinide. Unrecognised and potentially hazardous interaction between gemfibrozil and repaglinide should be considered. Concomitant use of gemfibrozil and repaglinide is best avoided. If the combination is considered necessary, repaglinide dosage should be greatly reduced and blood glucose concentrations carefully monitored [13].

Gemfibrozil and Glimepiride

Gemfibrozil increased the mean total area under the plasma concentration-time curve of glimepiride by 23%. No statistically significant differences were found in the serum insulin or blood glucose variables between the two phases. Gemfibrozil modestly increases the plasma concentrations of glimepiride. This may be caused by inhibition of CYP2C9 [14].

Gemfibrozil and Anticoaugulants

Potentiation of coumarin-type anti-coagulants has been observed with prolongation of the prothrombin time/INR when anti-coaugulants are administred in conjunction with gemfibrozil.

HIGHLIGHTS

Interactions between gemfibrozil and statins have been widely reported. Gemfibrozil can also potentially interact with some oral hypoglycemic agents, such as repaglinide and glimepiride prolonging the blood glucose-lowering effect. No interactions with ezetimibe have been described..

References

[1] Wen X, Wang JS, Backman JT, Kivisto KT, Neuvonen PJ Gemfibrozil is a potent inhibitor of human cytochrome P450 2C9. *Drug Metab Dispos.* 2001 Nov;29(11):1359-61.

[2] Pierce LR, Wysowski DK, Gross TP. Myopathy and rhabdomyolysis associated with lovastatin/gemfibrozil combination therapy. *JAMA* 1990;264:71-75.

[3] Bermingham RP, Whitsitt TB, Smart ML et al. Rhabdomyolysis in a patient receiving the combination of cerivastatin and gemfibrozil. Am J Health-Syst Pharm 2000;57:461-464.

[4] Duell PB, Connor WE, Illingworth DR. Rhabdomyolysis after taking atorvastatin with gemfibrozil. *Am J Cardiol* 1998;81:368-369.

[5] Tal A, Rajeshawari M, Isley W. Rhabdomyolysis associated with simvastatin/ gemfibrozil therapy. *South Med J* 1997;90:546-547.

[6] Prueksaritanont T, Zhao JJ, Ma B, Roadcap BA, Tang C, Qiu Y, Liu L, Lin JH, Pearson PG, Baillie TA Mechanistic studies on metabolic interactions between gemfibrozil and statins. *J Pharmacol Exp Ther.* 2002 Jun;301(3):1042-51.

[7] Walsky RL, Gaman EA, Obach RS. Examination of 209 drugs for inhibition of cytochrome P450 2C8. *J Clin Pharmacol* 2005; 45: 68–78.

[8] Shitara Y, Hirano M, Sato H, Sugiyama Y. Gemfibrozil and its glucuronide inhibit the organic anion transporting polypeptide 2 (OATP2/OATP1B1:SLC21A6)-mediated hepatic uptake and CYP2C8-mediated metabolism of cerivastatin: analysis of the mechanism of the clinically relevant drug-drug interaction between cerivastatin and gemfibrozil. *J Pharmacol Exp Ther.* 2004 Oct;311(1):228-36.

[9] Ballantyne CM, Davidson MH Possible differences between fibrates in pharmacokinetic interactions with statins. *Arch Intern Med.* 2003 Oct 27;163(19):2394-5.

[10] Martin PD, Dane AL, Schneck DW, Warwick MJ. An open-label, randomized, three-way crossover trial of the effects of coadministration of rosuvastatin and fenofibrate on the pharmacokinetic properties of rosuvastatin and fenofibric acid in healthy male volunteers. *Clin Ther.* 2003;25:459-471.

[11] Kyrklund C, Backman JT, Kivisto KT, Neuvonen M, Laitila J, Neuvonen PJ Plasma concentrations of active lovastatin acid are markedly increased by gemfibrozil but not by bezafibrate. *Clin Pharmacol Ther.* 2001 May;69(5):340-5.

[12] Reyderman L, Kosoglou T, Statkevich P, Pember L, Boutros T, Maxwell SE, Affrime M, Batra V. Assessment of a multiple-dose drug interaction between ezetimibe, a novel selective cholesterol absorption inhibitor and gemfibrozil. *Int J Clin Pharmacol Ther.* 2004 Sep;42(9):512-8.

[13] Niemi M, Backman JT, Neuvonen M, Neuvonen PJ. Effects of gemfibrozil, itraconazole, and their combination on the pharmacokinetics and pharmacodynamics of repaglinide: potentially hazardous interaction between gemfibrozil and repaglinide. *Diabetologia.* 2003 Mar;46:347-51.

[14] Niemi M, Neuvonen PJ, Kivisto KT Effect of gemfibrozil on the pharmacokinetics and pharmacodynamics of glimepiride. *Clin Pharmacol Ther.* 2001 Nov;70(5):439-45.

FENOFIBRATE

Brief Compound Description

The chemical name for fenofibrate is 2-[4-(4-chlorobenzoyl) phenoxy]-2-methyl-propanoic acid, 1-methylethyl ester. The empirical formula is C 20 H 21 O 4 Cl. Fenofibrate has the following structural formula:

Drug Interactions

Main of the possible drug-drug interactions between Fenofibrate and other components used in patients with metabolic syndrome are summarized in Table 1. The mechanisms and some of these potential interactions are discussed in detail below.

Table 1. Potential drug-drug interactions with fenofibrate in metabolic syndrome

YES	Mechanism and effect	NO	Potential
Warfarin	⇒ prolongation of the prothrombin time/INR	Simvastatin Pravastatin Repaglinide	Ezetimibe ○
Resins	⇓ reduced absorption of fenofibrate		

○ reported to be clinically not relevant.

Fenofibrate and HMG-CoA Reductase Inhibitors

The combined use of fenofibrate and HMG-CoA reductase inhibitors should be avoided unless the benefit of further alterations in lipid levels is likely to outweigh the increased risk of this drug combination. In a single-dose drug interaction study in 23 healthy adults the concomitant administration of fenofibrate and pravastatin resulted in no clinically important difference in the pharmacokinetics of fenofibric acid, pravastatin or its active metabolite 3(alpha)-hydroxy isopravastatin when compared to either drug given alone.

Similarly, no clinically significant pharmacokinetic drug interaction between fenofibrate and simvastatin was concluded in humans [1].

Fenofibrate and Resins

Bile acid sequestrants have been shown to bind other drugs given concurrently. Therefore, fenofibrate should be taken at least 1 hour before or 4 to 6 hours after a bile acid binding resin to avoid impeding its absorption.

Fenofibrate and Repaglinide

Bezafibrate and fenofibrate do not affect the pharmacokinetics or pharmacodynamics of repaglinide [2].

Fenofibrate and Ezetimibe

Ezetimibe did not significantly affect the pharmacokinetics of fenofibrate. Concomitant fenofibrate administration significantly increased the mean C(max) and AUC of total ezetimibe approximately 64% and 48%, respectively. However, based on the established safety profile and flat dose-response of ezetimibe, this effect is not considered to be clinically significant [3].

Fenofibrate and Anticoaugulants

The addition of fenofibrate in 2 patients on stable and therapeutic doses of warfarin increased the anticoagulant response to warfarin. A clear temporal relationship with the addition of fenofibrate and the appearance of the interaction was seen. Fenofibrate is highly protein bound, with the potential to displace warfarin from its binding protein, leading to an enhanced hypoprothrombinemic effect. Fenofibrate is also a mild to moderate inhibitor of CYP2C9, the enzyme responsible for warfarin metabolism. The combination of these effects--displacement of warfarin by fenofibrate coupled with decreased metabolism of warfarin--may increase the anticoagulant response to warfarin. Using the Naranjo probability scale, these interactions were designated as probable [4-6].

References

[1] Bergman AJ, Murphy G, Burke J, Zhao JJ, Valesky R, Liu L, Lasseter KC, He W, Prueksaritanont T, Qiu Y, Hartford A, Vega JM, Paolini JFSimvastatin does not have a clinically significant pharmacokinetic interaction with fenofibrate in humans. *J Clin Pharmacol.* 2004 Sep;44(9):1054-62.

[2] Kajosaari LI, Backman JT, Neuvonen M, Laitila J, Neuvonen PJ Lack of effect of bezafibrate and fenofibrate on the pharmacokinetics and pharmacodynamics of repaglinide. *Br J Clin Pharmacol.* 2004 Oct;58(4):390-6.

[3] Kosoglou T, Statkevich P, Fruchart JC, Pember LJ, Reyderman L, Cutler DL, Guillaume M, Maxwell SE, Veltri EP Pharmacodynamic and pharmacokinetic interaction between fenofibrate and ezetimibe. *Curr Med Res Opin.* 2004 Aug;20(8):1197-207.

[4] Kim KY, Mancano MA Fenofibrate potentiates warfarin effects. *Ann Pharmacother.* 2003 Feb;37(2):212-5.

[5] Ascah KJ, Rock GA, Wells PS. *Interaction between fenofibrate and warfarin.Ann Pharmacother.* 1998 Jul-Aug;32(7-8):765-8.

[6] Aldridge MA, Ito MK Fenofibrate and warfarin interaction. *Pharmacotherapy.* 2001 Jul;21(7):886-9.

NICOTINIC ACID (NIACIN)

Brief Compound Description

Nicotinic acid (Niacin) is a member of the B-vitamin family. Molecular formula:C6H4NO2CL; Molecular weight:157.5 The structural formula is the following:

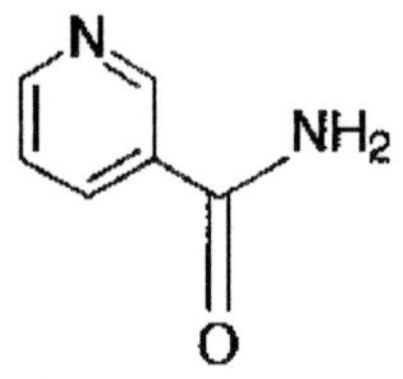

Mechanism of Action

Nicotinic acid lowers serum levels of total cholesterol, low-density lipoprotein cholesterol (LDL-C), very low-density lipoprotein (VLDL) and triglycerides. High-dose nicotinic acid also increases serum levels of high-density lipoprotein cholesterol (HDL-C) and decreases serum levels of lipoprotein (a) [Lp(a] and apolipoprotein B-100 (Apo B). The mechanism of the antihyperlipidemic action of nicotinic acid is not well understood. It is thought that this effect is mediated, in part, via decreases in the release of free fatty acids from adipose tissue, thereby decreasing the influx of free fatty acids into the liver, the hepatic reesterification of free fatty acids and the rate of production of hepatic very low-density lipoprotein (VLDL). A decrease in the hepatic production of VLDL reduces the level of circulating VLDL available for conversion to LDL. Another hypothesis holds that nicotinic acid directly inhibits hepatic synthesis or secretion of apolipoprotein B-containing lipoproteins. Still another hypothesis holds that nicotinic acid has the potential to cause a generalized inhibition of synthetic function in the liver. This mechanism may be considered a manifestation of nicotinic acid hepatotoxicity resulting in decreased LDL-cholesterol. However, this liver-damaging hypothesis would not explain the HDL-elevating effect of nicotinic acid. The mechanism by which nicotinic acid elevates HDL is unknown.High dose nicotinic acid has been found to significantly decrease cardiovascularand cerebrovascular events in those with coronary heart disease. It is thought that this effect is due, in part, to nicotinic acid's antihyperlipidemic activity [1-2].

Drug Interactions

Main of the possible drug-drug interactions between Nicotinc acid (niacin) and other components used in patients with metabolic syndrome are summarized in Table 1. The mechanisms and some of these potential interactions are discussed in detail below.

Nicotinic Acid and Calcium Channel Blockers

Concomitant use of high-dose nicotinic acid and a calcium channel blocker may potentiate the hypotensive effect of the calcium channel blocker

Nicotinic Acid and Alpha-glucosidase Inhibitors (Acarbose, Miglitol)

High-dose nicotinic acid may antagonize the antidiabetic action of alpha-glucosidase inhibitors, requiring adjustment of their dosage.

Table 1. Potential drug-drug interactions with Nicotinc acid (niacin) in metabolic syndrome

YES	Mechanism and effect
Alpha1-blockers Calcium channel blockers Nitrates	↑ increased concentration, increased hypotensive effect
Alpha-glucosidase inhibitors Metformin Sulfonylureas Repaglinide Glitazones	↓ decreased concentration, decreased hypoglycemic effect
Statins Gemfibrozil Cholestyramine Colestipol	↔complementary antihyperlipidemic effects
Warfarin	⇒ prolongation of the prothrombin time/INR

Nicotinic Acid and Metformin

High-dose nicotinic acid may antagonize the antidiabetic activity of metformin, requiring adjustment of its dosage.

Nicotinic Acid and Cholestyramine

Concomitant use of high-dose nicotinic acid and cholestyramine may reduce the absorption of nicotinic acid. It is recommended that a 4 to 6 hour interval elapse between the ingestion of cholestyramine and the administration of nicotinic acid. Administration of high-dose nicotinic acid and cholestyramine may produce complementary antihyperlipidemic effects.

Nicotinic Acid and Colestipol

Concomitant use of high-dose nicotinic acid and colestipol may reduce the absorption of nicotinic acid. It is recommended that a 4 to 6 hour interval elapse between the ingestion of colestipol and the administration of nicotinic acid. Administraion of high-dose nicotinic acid and colestipol may produce complementary antihyperlipidemic effects.

Nicotinic Acid and Gemfibrozil

Adminisration of high-dose nicotinic acid and gemfibrozil may produce complementary antihyperlipidemic effects.

Nicotinic Acid and Statins

Concomitant administration of high-dose nicotinic acid and HMG-CoA reductase inhibitors have resulted in rare cases of rhabdomyolysis. Those receiving concomitant high-dose nicotinic acid and an HMG-CoA reductase inhibitor should be carefully monitored for any signs or symptoms of muscle pain, tenderness or weakness. Administration of high-dose nicotinic acid and a statin may produce complementary antihyperlipidemic effects.

Nicotinic Acid and Repaglinide

High-dose nicotinic acid may antagonize the antidiabetic action of repaglinide, a metglitinide analogue, requiring adjustment of its dosage.

Nicotinic Acid and Nicotine Patch

Concomitant use of a transdermal nicotine patch and nicotinic acid may enhance the flushing reaction.

Nicotinic acid and Nitrates

Concomitant use of high-dose nicotinic acid and a nitrate may potentiate the hypotensive effect of the nitrate.

Nicotinic Acid and NSAIDs (Ibuprofen, etc.) and Aspirin

The use of aspirin, ibuprofen, or other NSAIDs, taken 30 minutes to one hour before a dose of nicotinic acid, may blunt the flushing effect of high-dose nicotinic acid. Nicotinic acid induces the release of prostacyclin. Prostacyclin is thought to account for, in large part, nicotinic acid-induced flushing. Aspirin may also decrease the metabolic clearance of nicotinic acid.

Nicotinic Acid and Sulfonylureas (Chlorpropamide, Glimepiride, Glipizide, Glyburide)

High-dose nicotinic acid may antagonize the antidiabetic action of sulfonylureas, requiring adjustment of their dosage.

Nicotinic Acid and Thiazolidinediones (Pioglitazone, Rosiglitazone)

High-dose nicotinic acid may antagonize the antidiabetic action of thiazolidinediones, requiring adjustment of their dosage.

Nicotinic Acid and Warfarin

Extended-release (intermediate-release) forms of nicotinic acid have been associated with small but statistically significant increases in prothrombin time. Concomitant use of extended-release forms of nicotinic acid, as well as other forms of nicotinic acid, may enhance the anticoagulant activity of warfarin. INRs should be closely monitored in those taking high-dose nicotinic acid concomitantly with warfarin.

References

[1] Goldberg A, Alagona P Jr, Capuzzi DM, et al. Multiple-dose efficacy and safety of an extended-release form of niacin in the management of hyperlipidemia. *Am J Cardiol.* 2000; 85:1100-1105.

[2] Capuzzi DM, Guyton JR, Morgan JM, et al. Efficacy and safety of an extended-release niacin (Niaspan): a long-term study. *Am J Cardiol.* 1998; 82(12A):74U-81U.

PROBUCOL

Brief Compound Description

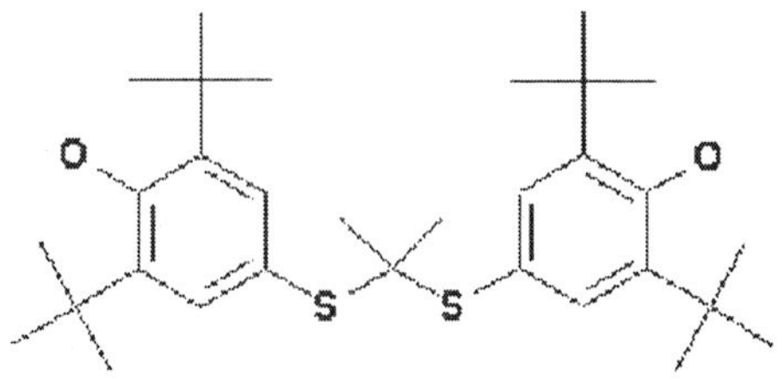

Probucol

Mechanism of Action

Probucol increases the rate of LDL metabolism and may block the intestinal transport of cholesterol. The net result is a significant reduction in plasma cholesterol levels.

Drug Interactions

The effects of probucol, a cholesterol-lowering agent, on several cytochrome P450 (CYP) isoform-specific reactions in human liver microsomes were investigated to predict drug interactions with probucol in vivo from in vitro data. Probucol had neither stimulatory nor inhibitory effects on CYP1Al/2, 2A6, 2B6, 2C8/9, 2C19, 2D6, 2E1, and 3A4 activities at concentrations up to 300 microM, indicating that probucol, at the expected therapeutic concentrations, would not be predicted to cause clinically significant interactions with other CYP-metabolized drugs [1].

Probucol may have potential drug interactions with antidysrhythmics. The major interaction involving probucol is a possible additive effect with drugs or clinical conditions that alter the prolongation of the QTc interval, increasing the potential for polymorphic ventricular tachycardia, such as torsade de pointes [2-3]. Probucol is known to induce QT prolongation in some patients, although ventricular arrhythmia or syncope due to the drug is rare [4].

References

[1] Umehara K, Shimokawa Y, Miyamoto G Effect of probucol on cytochrome P450 activities in human liver microsomes.*Biol Pharm Bull.* 2002 Aug;25(8):1112-4.

[2] Farmer JA, Gotto AM Jr Antihyperlipidaemic agents. Drug interactions of clinical significance. *Drug Saf.* 1994 Nov;11(5):301-9.

[3] Ohya, Y., Kumamoto, K., Abe, I., Tsubota, Y, Fujishima, M. Factors related to QT interval prolongation during probucol treatment. *Eur. J. Clin. Pharmacol.* 1993;45: 47–52.

[4] Hayashik et al. Probucol aggravates long QT syndrome associated with a novel missense mutation M124T in the N-terminus of HERG *Clinical Science* 2004; 107:175–182.

CHOLESTYRAMINE

Brief Compound Description

Cholestyramine is the chloride salt of a basic anion exchange resin. The structural formula is the following:

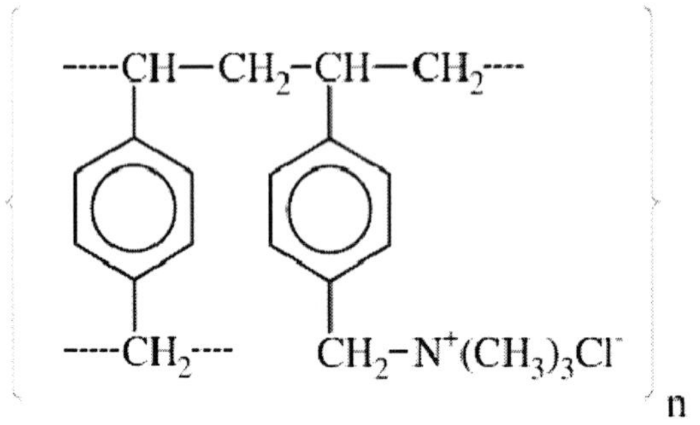

$-CH-CH_2-CH-CH_2-$

$-CH_2-$ $CH_2-N^+(CH_3)_3Cl^-$

n

CHOLESTYRAMINE

Mechanism of Action

Bile acid resins absorb bile acid in the intestinal tract rather than letting it be reabsorbed and reused by the body. This bile deficit causes the liver to produce more bile. Since the liver uses cholesterol to produce bile, bile acid resins reduce cholesterol levels in the blood stream.

Drug Interactions

Cholestyramine decreases the absorption of warfarin, thyroid hormones, digoxin, thiazide diuretics and glitazones. Therefore, these drugs should be administered 1 hour before or 4-6 hours after the administration of cholestyramine. Cholestyramine decreases the oral absorption of many concurrently administered drugs, including NSAIDs [1].

Cholestyramine and Thyroid Hormones

Cholestyramine has been shown to bind thyroid hormones in the intestine, reducing absorption of these agents. This interaction can be minimized, but not necessarily avoided, by separating the administration of cholestyramine and thyroid replacement products by six hours, and by consistently administering the medications the same number of hours apart every day. Since enterohepatic circulation of thyroid hormones may contribute to this interaction, as with oral anticoagulants, this interaction may not be completely avoided by separating doses [2].

References

[1] Verbeeck RK Pharmacokinetic drug interactions with nonsteroidal anti-inflammatory drugs. *Clin Pharmacokinet.* 1990 Jul;19(1):44-66.

[2] Kastrup EK. *Drug Facts and Comparisons. Facts and Comparisons,* St. Louis, MO. 2000.

EZETIMIBE

Brief Compound Description

Ezetimibe is in a class of lipid-lowering compounds that selectively inhibits the intestinal absorption of cholesterol and related phytosterols. The chemical name of ezetimibe is 1-(4-fluorophenyl)-3(R)-[3-(4-fluorophenyl)-3(S)-hydroxypropyl]-4(S)-(4-hydroxyphenyl)-2-azetidinone. The empirical formula is $C_{24}H_{21}F_2NO_3$. Its molecular weight is 409.4 and its structural formula is:

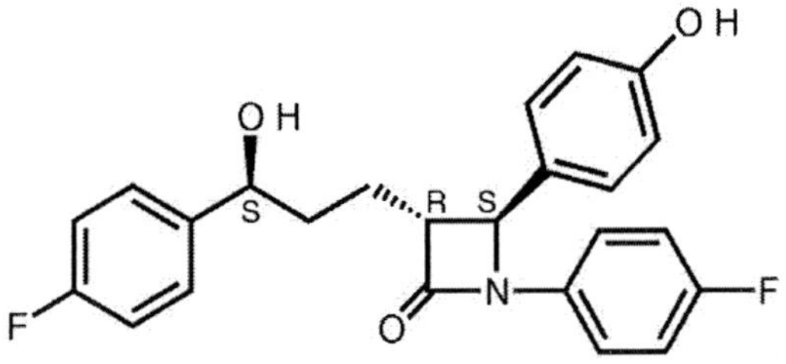

Mechanism of Action

Ezetimibe is the first agent of a novel class of selective cholesterol absorption inhibitors recently approved by the Food and Drug Administration for treatment in the United States. Ezetimibe inhibits the absorption of biliary and dietary cholesterol from the small intestine without affecting the absorption of fat-soluble vitamins, triglycerides, or bile acids. Ezetimibe localizes at the brush border of the small intestine and decreases cholesterol uptake into the enterocytes [1-2].

Drug Interactions

Ezetimibe has no significant effect on a series of probe drugs known to be metabolized by cytochrome P450. This indicates that ezetimibe is neither an inhibitor nor an inducer of these cytochrome P450 isozymes, and it is unlikely that ezetimibe will affect the metabolism of drugs that are metabolized by these enzymes.

Main of the possible drug-drug interactions between ezetimibe and other components used in patients with metabolic syndrome are summarized in Table 1. The mechanisms and some of these potential interactions are discussed in detail below.

Table 1. Potential drug-drug interactions with ezetimibe in metabolic syndrome

YES	Mechanism and effect	NO	Potential
Gemfibrozil	⇑ increased concentration of ezetimibe	Statins Glipizide Digoxin	Fenofibrate ○
Cholestyramine	⇓ decreased absorption of ezetimibe	Warfarin Oral Contraceptives	

○ reported to be clinically not relevant

Ezetimibe and Statins

In studies of healthy hypercholesterolemic adult subjects, concomitant administration of ezetimibe (10 mg once daily) had no significant effect on the bioavailability of either lovastatin, simvastatin, pravastatin, atorvastatin, fluvastatin or rosuvastatin [4-7]. However, there is as yet no evidence that ezetimibe, when added to statin, increases the risk for myotoxicity or tendinopathy. This interaction, if present, has no known underlying mechanism. Candidate sites of pharmacokinetic interactions might be glucuronidation —both ezetimibe and atorvastatin, but not fluvastatin, undergo glucuronidation—or organic anion transporting polypeptide type 2 (OATP2) (mediating hepatic uptake), of which several statins are substrates. This interaction may be important because ezetimibe is usually prescribed in combination [8].

Ezetimibe and Gemfibrozil

Concomitant administration of gemfibrozil (600 mg twice daily) significantly increased the oral bioavailability of total ezetimibe by a factor of 1.7. Ezetimibe (10 mg once daily) did not significantly affect the bioavailability of gemfibrozil.

Ezetimibe and Fenofibrate

In a study of healthy hypercholesterolemic adult subjects, concomitant fenofibrate (200 mg once daily) administration increased the mean C max and AUC values of total ezetimibe approximately 64% and 48%, respectively. Pharmacokinetics of fenofibrate were not significantly affected by ezetimibe (10 mg once daily) [9].

Ezetimibe and Cholestyramine

In a study of healthy hypercholesterolemic adult subjects, concomitant cholestyramine (4 g twice daily) administration decreased the mean AUC values of total ezetimibe and ezetimibe approximately 55% and 80%, respectively.

Ezetimibe and Warfarin

Concomitant administration of ezetimibe (10 mg once daily) had no significant effect on bioavailability of warfarin and prothrombin time.

Ezetimibe and Digoxin

Concomitant administration of ezetimibe (10 mg once daily) had no significant effect on the bioavailability of digoxin and the ECG parameters (HR, PR, QT, and QTc intervals) in a study of twelve healthy adult males.

Ezetimibe and Oral Contraceptives

Co-administration of ezetimibe (10 mg once daily) with oral contraceptives had no significant effect on the bioavailability of ethinyl estradiol or levonorgestrel.

Ezetimibe and Cimetidine

Multiple doses of cimetidine (400 mg twice daily) had no significant effect on the oral bioavailability of ezetimibe and total ezetimibe.

Ezetimibe and Glipizide

Steady-state levels of ezetimibe (10 mg once daily) had no significant effect on the pharmacokinetics and pharmacodynamics of glipizide. A single dose of glipizide (10 mg) had no significant effect on the exposure to total ezetimibe or ezetimibe.

HIGHLIGHTS

Ezetimibe can be safely co-administred with most of other drugs used for the treatment of patients with metabolic syndrome. However a potential interaction with fibrates occurs, but it seems to be clinically not relevant..

References

[1] Bays HE, Moore PB, Drehobl MA, Rosenblatt S, Toth PD, Dujovne CA, et al.Effectiveness and tolerability of ezetimibe in patients with primary hypercholesterolemia:pooled analysis of two phase II studies. *Clin Ther.* 2001;23:1209-30.

[2] Kosoglou T, Statkevich P, Yang B, Suresh R, Zhu Y, Boutros T, Maxwell SE, Tiessen R, Cutler DL. Pharmacodynamic interaction between ezetimibe and rosuvastatin. *Curr Med Res Opin.* 2004 Aug;20(8):1185-95.

[3] Gagne C, Gaudet D, Bruckert E. Efficacy and safety of ezetimibe coadministered with atorvastatin or simvastatin in patients with homozygous familial hypercholesterolemia. *Circulation.* 2002;105:2469-75.

[4] Davidson MH, McGarry T, Bettis R, Melani L, Lipka LJ, LeBeaut AP, et al.*Ezetimibe coadministered with simvastatin in patients with primary hypercholesterolemia.*

[5] Fux R, Morike K, Gundel UF, Hartmann R, Gleiter CH. Ezetimibe and statin-associated myopathy. *Ann Intern Med.* 2004 Apr 20;140(8):671-2.

[6] Ballantyne CM, Houri J, Notarbartolo A, Melani L, Lipka LJ, Suresh R, Sun S, LeBeaut AP, Sager PT, Veltri EP; Ezetimibe Study Group Effect of ezetimibe coadministered with atorvastatin in 628 patients with primary hypercholesterolemia: a prospective, randomized, double-blind trial. *Circulation.* 2003 May 20;107(19):2409-15.

[7] Patrick JE, Kosoglou T, Stauber KL, Alton KB, Maxwell SE, Zhu Y, et al. Disposition of the selective cholesterol absorption inhibitor ezetimibe in healthy male subjects. *Drug Metab Dispos.* 2002;30:430-7.

[8] Prueksaritanont T, Subramanian R, Fang X, Ma B, Qiu Y, Lin JH, et al. Glucuronidation of statins in animals and humans: a novel mechanism of statin lactonization. *Drug Metab Dispos.* 2002;30:505-12.

[9] Reyderman L, Kosoglou T, Statkevich P, Pember L, Boutros T, Maxwell SE, Affrime M, Batra V. Pharmacodynamic and pharmacokinetic interaction between fenofibrate and ezetimibe. *Curr Med Res Opin.* 2004 Aug;20(8):1197-207.

Chapter 5

ANTI-HYPERTENSIVE DRUGS

CALCIUM CHANNEL BLOCKING AGENTS (CA ANTAGONISTS)

Verapamil

Brief Compound Description

Verapamil [2, 8-bis-(3, 4-dimethoxyphenyl)-6-methyl-2-isopropyl-6-azaoctanitrile] is a calcium channel blocking agent used in the treatment of various cardiovascular disorders. Verapamil undergoes extensive hepatic first pass metabolism

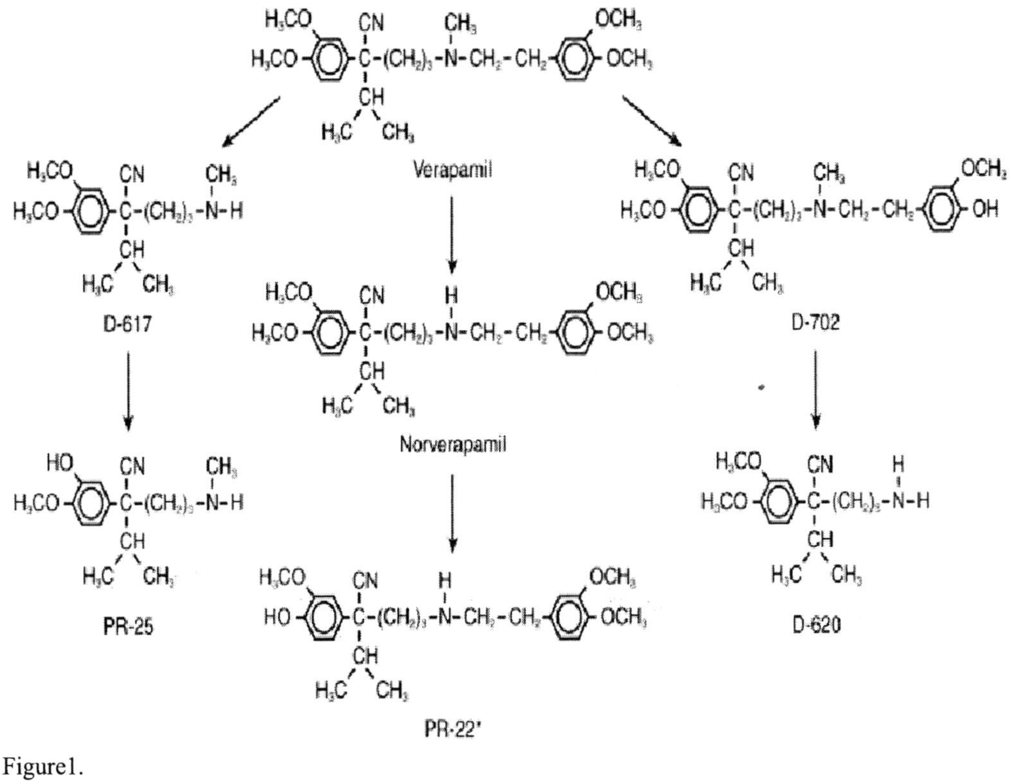

Figure1.

Structures of verapamil and its primary metabolites indicating the major routes of oxidative metabolism. from *Tracy TS, et al. Cytochrome P450 isoforms involved in metabolism of the enantiomers of verapamil and norverapamil. Br J Clin Pharmacol. 1999 May;47(5):545-52.*

Mechanism of Action

Verapamil is a calcium ion influx inhibitor. The mechanism of the antianginal and antiarrhythmic effects of verapamil is believed to be related to its specific cellular action of selectively inhibiting transmembrane influx of calcium in cardiac muscle, coronary and systemic arteries and in cells of the intracardiac conduction system. Verapamil blocks the transmembrane influx of calcium through the slow channel (calcium ion antagonism) without affecting, to any significant degree the transmembrane influx of sodium through the fast channel. This results in a reduction of free calcium ions available within cells of the above tissues. Verapamil's antiarrhythmic effects are believed to be brought about largely by its action on the sinoatrial (SA) and atrioventricular (AV) nodes. Verapamil depresses AV nodal conduction and prolongs functional refractory periods. Verapamil does not alter the normal atrial action potential or intraventricular conduction time, but depresses amplitude, velocity of depolarization and conduction in depressed atrial fibers.

Drug Interactions

Data suggest that P450s 3A4, 3A5 and 2C8 are the predominant isoforms involved in the metabolism of R- and S-verapamil as well as R- and S-norverapamil. Compounds interfering with cytochromes P450 3A4 and 3A5 can potentially cause drug interactions when given with verapamil, particularly in light of the roles P450 3A4 and 3A5 play in both presystemic and hepatic drug metabolism.

Clinically important mechanism-based CYP3A4 inhibitors include antihypertensives (e.g. dihydralazine, verapamil and diltiazem) [1]. Genetic studies seem to indicate that the presence of variable CYP3A5/CYP3A4 expression in the liver may contribute to the interindividual variability associated with verapamil mediated drug interactions [2].

Verapamil and Statins

Studies compared the multiple-dose pharmacokinetic interaction profiles of pravastatin, simvastatin, and atorvastatin when coadministered with verapamil in healthy subjects. Concomitant verapamil increased the simvastatin area under the concentration:time curve (AUC) approximately fourfold, the maximum serum concentration (C(max)) fivefold, and the active metabolite simvastatin acid AUC and C(max) approximately four- and threefold, respectively [3-4]. These data could suggest that concomitant use of verapamil and simvastatin should be avoided or the simvastatin dosage should be markedly decreased (50% to 80%)

Verapamil and Beta-Adrenergic Blockers

Potential pharmacodynamic and pharmacokinetic interactions between verapamil and propranolol have been suggested [5]. Verapamil increased the AUC and Cmax and shortened the tmax of propranolol. Propranolol decreased the AUC and Cmax of verapamil. The greater reduction of heart rate with the combination of verapamil and propranolol was only partially explained by higher plasma concentrations of propranolol. The combination of propranolol and verapamil produced clinically important synergistic adverse effects during exercise. Negative dromotropic effects occurred primarily by direct AV node inhibition and were more important than previously recognized [6].

Although repeated administration of propranolol reduced hepatic blood flow as assessed by indocyanine green clearance, there was no evidence of an interaction between the drugs at this level. Some studies showed that the pharmacokinetics of verapamil and norverapamil were not significantly affected by prior propranolol. After single doses of verapamil and propranolol in combination, the maximum plasma concentration of propranolol was increased and the oral clearance of verapamil reduced. No pharmacokinetic interaction was observed after repeated doses. Few evidences of a pharmacodynamic or pharmacokinetic interaction between verapamil and propranolol in normal subjects occur. Most of the haemodynamic responses to these drugs in combination can be explained by additive drug effects but an interaction affecting AV conduction after repeated doses cannot be excluded. The minor pharmacokinetic interaction between the drugs is unlikely to be relevant to the pharmacodynamic changes [7].

Verapamil and Digoxin

Verapamil has been demonstrated to inhibit the elimination of digoxin and to increase its steady state plasma level by 60-80%. The main inhibitory effect of verapamil on digoxin elimination is on the biliary route [8] Verapamil treatment increases serum digoxin levels by 50 to 75% during the first week of therapy, and this can result in digitalis toxicity. In patients with hepatic cirrhosis the influence of verapamil on digoxin kinetics is magnified. Verapamil may reduce total body clearance and extrarenal clearance of digoxin by 27 and 29% respectively. Maintenance and digitalization doses should be reduced when verapamil is administered and the patient should be reassessed to avoid over- or underdigitalization. Whenever overdigitalization is suspected, the daily dose of digitalis should be reduced or temporarily discontinued. On discontinuation of verapamil use, the patient should be reassessed to avoid underdigitalization [9].

Verapamil and Antiarrhythmic Agents

Quinidine

In a small number of patients with hypertrophic cardiomyopathy, concomitant use of verapamil and quinidine resulted in significant hypotension. Verapamil significantly counteracted the effects of quinidine on AV conduction. There has been a report of increased quinidine levels during verapamil therapy.

Disopyramide

Until data on possible interactions between verapamil and disopyramide are obtained, disopyramide should not be administered within 48 hours before or 24 hours after verapamil administration.

Flecainide

A study in healthy volunteers showed that the concomitant administration of flecainide and verapamil may have additive effects on myocardial contractility, AV conduction, and repolarization. Concomitant therapy with flecainide and verapamil may result in additive negative inotropic effect and prolongation of atrioventricular conduction.

Dofetilide

Potential kinetic and dynamic interactions between the new class III antiarrhythmic dofetilide and the calcium channel blocker verapamil have been evaluated. The maximal mean increase in QT, over steady-state baseline values was 20 msec for dofetilide alone versus 26 msec during combination therapy. This relatively small interactive effect occurred only while peak plasma drug concentrations were developing at 1 to 3 hours after dosing and is probably caused by the known effect of verapamil to increase hepatic and portal bloodflow. According to this interaction and the relationship between dofetilide plasma concentration and torsade, verapamil is contraindicated in patients receiving dofetilide [10].

Verapamil and Nitrates, Diuretics

No cardiovascular adverse effects have been attributed to any interaction between these agents and verapamil.

Verapamil and Cimetidine

Controversial data on the possible intreaction between verapamil and cimtidine. In fact, two clinical trials have shown a lack of significant verapamil interaction with cimetidine, whereas a third study showed cimetidine reduced verapamil clearance and increased elimination half-life.

HIGHLIGHTS

Verapamil has the potentiality to interact with statins, beta-blockers and digoxin.

References

[1] Zhou S, Yung Chan S, Cher Goh B, Chan E, Duan W, Huang M, McLeod HLMechanism-Based Inhibition of Cytochrome P450 3A4 by Therapeutic Drugs. *Clin Pharmacokinet. 2005*;44(3):279-304.

[2] Wang YH, Jones DR, Hall SD. Differential mechanism-based inhibition of CYP3A4 by verapamil. *Drug Metab Dispos.* 2005 Feb 2.

[3] Jacobson TA Comparative pharmacokinetic interaction profiles of pravastatin, simvastatin, and atorvastatin when coadministered with cytochrome P450 inhibitors. *Am J Cardiol.* 2004 Nov 1;94(9):1140-6.

[4] Kantola, T., Kivisto, K.T., Neuvonen, P.J.. Erythromycin and verapamil considerably increase serum simvastatin and simvastatin acid concentrations, *Clin Pharmacol Ther* 1998; 64: 177–182.

[5] Bauer LA, Horn JR, Maxon MS, Easterling TR, Shen DD, Strandness DE JrEffect of metoprolol and verapamil administered separately and concurrently after single doses on liver blood flow and drug disposition. *J Clin Pharmacol.* 2000 May;40(5):533-43.

[6] Carruthers SG, Freeman DJ, Bailey DG. Synergistic adverse hemodynamic interaction between oral verapamil and propranolol. *Clin Pharmacol Ther* 1989;46:469-77.

[7] Murdoch DL, Thomson GD, Thompson GG, Murray GD, Brodie MJ, McInnes GT. Evaluation of potential pharmacodynamic and pharmacokinetic interactions between verapamil and propranolol in normal subjects. *Br J Clin Pharmacol.* 1991 Mar;31(3):323-32.

[8] Hedman A, Angelin B, Arvidsson A, Beck O, Dahlqvist R, Nilsson B, Olsson M, Schenck-Gustafsson K. Digoxin-verapamil interaction: reduction of biliary but not renal digoxin clearance in humans. *Clin Pharmacol Ther.* 1991 Mar;49(3):256-62.

[9] Pedersen KE, Thayssen P, Klitgaard NA, Christiansen BD, Nielsen-Kudsk F. Influence of verapamil on the inotropism and pharmacokinetics of digoxin. *Eur J Clin Pharmacol.* 1983;25(2):199-206.

[10] Johnson, BF, Cheng, SL, and Venitz, J. Transient kinetic and dynamic interactions between verapamil and dofetilide, a class III antiarrhythmic. *Journal of Clinical Pharmacology,* 2001; 41:1248-1256.

DILTIAZEM

Brief Compound Description

Diltiazem HCl is a calcium ion influx inhibitor (slow channel blocker or calcium antagonist). Chemically, diltiazem HCL is 1,5-benzothiazepin-4(5H)one, 3- (acetyloxy)-5-[2-(dimethylamino) ethyl]-2, 3-dihydro-2-(4-methoxyphenyl)-, monohydrochloride, (+)-cis-.The structural formula is the following:

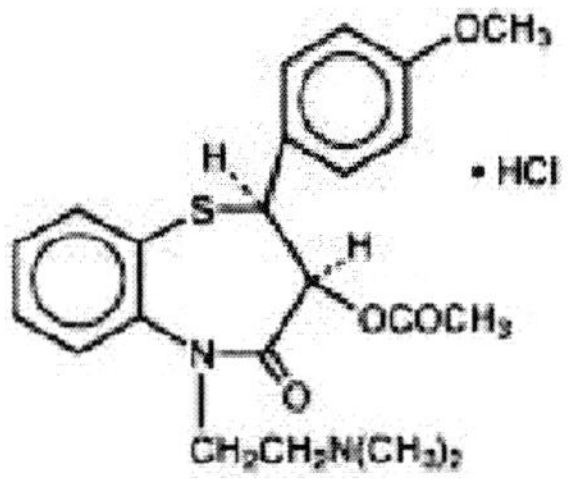

Drug Interactions

Diltiazem is extensively metabolized in the liver, primarily by deacetylation and demethylation by CYP3A4 into a host metabolite, N-desmethyl-diltiazem, which, together with diltiazem, in turn selectively inhibits CYP3A4, but not CYP1A2, CYP2C9, or CYP2E1 [1-2]. Accordingly, pharmacokinetic and pharmacodynamic interactions may theoretically happen upon co-administration of diltiazem and a drug metabolized by CYP3A4 like simvastatin.

Diltiazem and Statins

Combined treatment of diltiazem and simvastatin has been shown to cause a 5-fold increase in the AUC of simvastatin suggesting a pharmacokinetically-driven pharmacodynamic interaction between the two drugs [3-4]. Diltiazem coadministration resulted in a significant interaction with simvastatin, probably by inhibiting CYP3A-mediated metabolism. Concomitant use of diltiazem or other potent inhibitors of CYP3A with simvastatin should be avoided, or close clinical monitoring should be used [4 -5].

References

[1] D.R. Jones, J.C. Gorski, M.A. Hamman, B.S. Mayhew, S. Rider, S.D. Hall. Diltiazem inhibition of cytochrome P-450 3A activity is due to metabolite intermediate complex formation, *Journal of Pharmacology and Experimental Therapeutics* 1999; 290: 1116–1125.

[2] Sutton, A.M. Butler, L. Nadin, M. Murray. Role of CYP3A4 in human hepatic diltiazem N-demethylation: inhibition of CYP3A4 activity by oxidized diltiazem metabolites, *Journal of Pharmacology and Experimental Therapeutics* 1997;282: pp. 294–300.

[3] O. Mousa, D.C. Brater, K.J. Sunblad, S.D. Hall The interaction of diltiazem with simvastatin, *Clinical Pharmacology and Therapeutics* 2000;67: 267–274.

[4] N.E. Azie, D.C. Brater, P.A. Becker, D.R. Jones, S.D. Hall. The interaction of diltiazem with lovastatin and pravastatin, *Clinical Pharmacology and Therapeutics* 1998;64: 369–377.

[5] K.R. Yeo, W.W. Yeo, E.J. Wallis, L.E. Ramsay, Enhanced cholesterol reduction by simvastatin in diltiazem-treated patients, *British Journal of Clinical Pharmacology* 1999;48: 610–615.

[6] Watanabe H, Kosuge K, Nishio S, Yamada H, Uchida S, Satoh H, Hayashi H, Ishizaki T, Ohashi K Pharmacokinetic and pharmacodynamic interactions between simvastatin and diltiazem in patients with hypercholesterolemia and hypertension. *Life Sci.* 2004 Dec 3;76(3):281-92.

NIFEDIPINE

Brief Compound Description

Nifedipine is 3,5-pyridinedicarboxylic acid, 1,4-dihydro-2, 6-dimethyl-4-(2-nitrophenyl)-, dimethyl ester, C17H18N2O6, and has this structural formula:

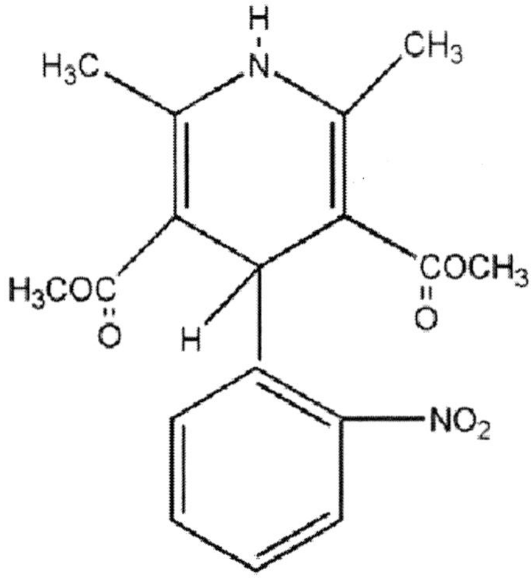

Mechanism of Action

Nifedipine is a calcium ion influx inhibitor (slow-channel blocker or calcium ion antagonist) and inhibits the transmembrane influx of calcium ions into cardiac muscle and smooth muscle. The contractile processes of cardiac muscle and vascular smooth muscle are dependent upon the movement of extracellular calcium ions into these cells through specific ion channels. Nifedipine selectively inhibits calcium ion influx across the cell membrane of cardiac muscle and vascular smooth muscle without changing serum calcium concentrations

Drug Interactions

Nifedipine and Beta Blocker

Combination of calcium-channel antagonists and ß-blockers may be synergistic in their negative effects on dromotropy, chronotropy, and inotropy. Coadministration of a ß-blocker with nifedipine may inhibit the compensatory sympathetic outflow normally seen in isolated nifedipine toxicity [1-3].

Nifedipine and Long-Acting Nitrates

nifedipine may be safely co-administered with nitrates, but there have been no controlled studies to evaluate the antianginal effectiveness of this combination.

Nifedipine and Digoxin

Since there have been isolated reports of patients with elevated digoxin levels, and there is a possible interaction between digoxin and nifedipine, it is recommended that digoxin levels be monitored when initiating, adjusting, and discontinuing nifedipine to avoid possible over- or under-digitalization.

Nifedipine and Quinidine

There have been rare reports of an interaction between quinidine and nifedipine (with a decreased plasma level of quinidine).

Nifedipine and Anticoagulants

There have been rare reports of increased prothrombin time in patients taking coumarin anticoagulants to whom nifedipine was administered.

References

[1] Schier JG, Howland MA, Hoffman RS, Nelson LS Fatality from administration of labetalol and crushed extended-release nifedipine. *Ann Pharmacother.* 2003 Oct;37(10):1420-3
[2] Piepho RW, Culbertson VL, Rhodes RS. Drug interactions with the calcium-entry blockers. *Circulation* 1987;75(suppl V):V -181-94.
[3] McAllister RG, Hamann SR, Blouin RA. Pharmacokinetics of calcium entry blockers. *Am J Cardiol* 1985;55:30B-40B.

AMLODIPINE

Brief Compound Description

Amlodipine is chemically described as (R.S.) 3-ethyl-5-methyl-2-(2-aminoethoxymethyl)-4-(2-chlorophenyl)-1,4-dihydro-6-methyl-3,5-pyridinedicarboxylate benzenesulphonate. Its empirical formula is C 20 H 25 CIN 2 O 5 ·C 6 H 6 O 3 S, and its structural formula is:

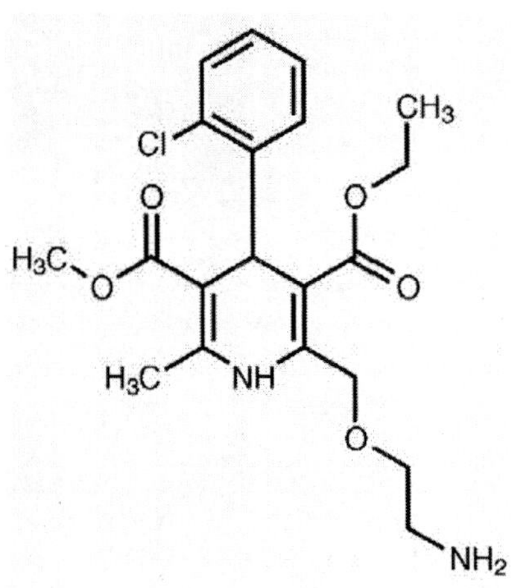

$C_6H_6O_3S$

Mechanism of Action

Amlodipine is a dihydropyridine calcium antagonist (calcium ion antagonist or slow-channel blocker) that inhibits the transmembrane influx of calcium ions into vascular smooth muscle and cardiac muscle. Experimental data suggest that Amlodipine binds to both dihydropyridine and nondihydropyridine binding sites. The contractile processes of cardiac muscle and vascular smooth muscle are dependent upon the movement of extracellular calcium ions into these cells through specific ion channels. Amlodipine inhibits calcium ion influx across cell membranes selectively, with a greater effect on vascular smooth muscle cells than on cardiac muscle cells.

Drug Interactions

Main of the possible drug-drug interactions between amlodipine and other components used in patients with metabolic syndrome are summarized in Table 1. The mechanisms and some of these potential interactions are discussed in detail below.

Table 1. Possible drug-drug interactions with amlodipine in metabolic syndrome

NO
Thiazide diuretics Beta-blockers ACE inhibitors Long-acting nitrates Sublingual nitroglycerin NASIDs Oral Hypoglycemic Drugs Atorvastatin Warfarin Digoxin Cimetidine

Amplodipine and Thiazide Diuretics, Beta-blockers, Angiotensin-converting Enzyme inhibitors, Long-acting Nitrates, Sublingual Nitroglycerin, Non-steroidal Anti-Inflammatory Drugs, and Oral Hypoglycemic Drugs

No interaction between amplodipine and these drugs have been reported.

Amplodipine and Atorvastatin

Co-administration of multiple 10 mg doses of Amplodipine with 80 mg of atorvastatin resulted in no significant change in the steady state pharmacokinetic parameters of atorvastatin.

Amplodipine and Digoxin

Co-administration of Amplodipine with digoxin did not change serum digoxin levels or digoxin renal clearance in normal volunteers.

Amplodipine and Alcohol

Single and multiple 10 mg doses of Amplodipine had no significant effect on the pharmacokinetics of ethanol.

Amplodipine and Warfarin

Co-administration of Amplodipine with warfarin did not change the warfarin prothrombin response time.

Amplodipine and Cimetidine

Co-administration of Amplodipine with cimetidine did not alter the pharmacokinetics of Amplodipine

Amplodipine and Sildenafil

A single 100 mg dose of sildenafil in subjects with essential hypertension had no effect on the pharmacokinetic parameters of Amplodipine

HIGHLIGHTS

Amlodipine can be safely co-administred with the majority of the drugs used for the treatment of patients with metabolic syndrome.

FELODIPINE

Brief Compound Description

Felodipine is a dihydropyridine derivative and optically active described as (¡Ó)ethyl methyl 4-(2,3-dichlorophenyl)-1,4-dihydro-2,6-dimethyl-3,5- pyridinedicarboxylate. Its empirical formula is C18H19Cl2NO4 with structural formula shown as

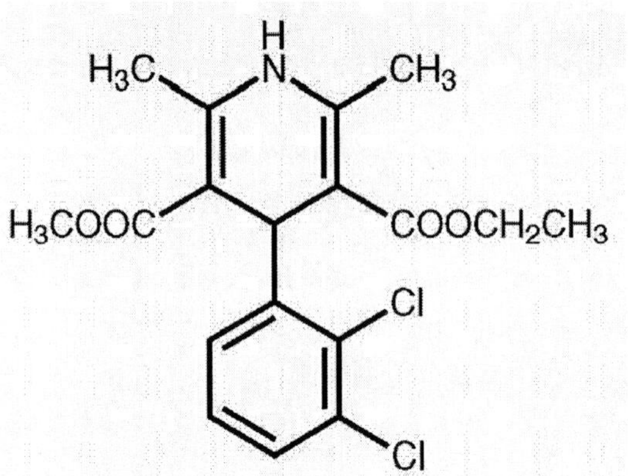

Drug Interactions

CYP3A4 Inhibitors --Felodipine is metabolized by CYP3A4. Co-administration of CYP3A4 inhibitors with felodipine may lead to several-fold increases in the plasma levels of felodipine, either due to an increase in bioavailability or due to a decrease in metabolism. These increases in concentration may lead to increased effects, lower blood pressure and increased heart rate.

Felodipine and Beta-blockers

A pharmacokinetic study of felodipine in conjunction with metoprolol demonstrated no significant effects on the pharmacokinetics of felodipine. The AUC and C max of metoprolol, however, were increased approximately 31% and 38%, respectively. In controlled clinical trials, however, beta blockers including metoprolol were concurrently administered with felodipine and were well tolerated.

NISOLDIPINE

Brief Compound Description

Nisoldipine is 3,5-pyridinedicarboxylic acid, 1,4-dihydro-2,6-dimethyl-4-(2-nitrophenyl)-, methyl 2-methylpropyl ester, C 20 H 24 N 2 O 6, and has the structural formula:

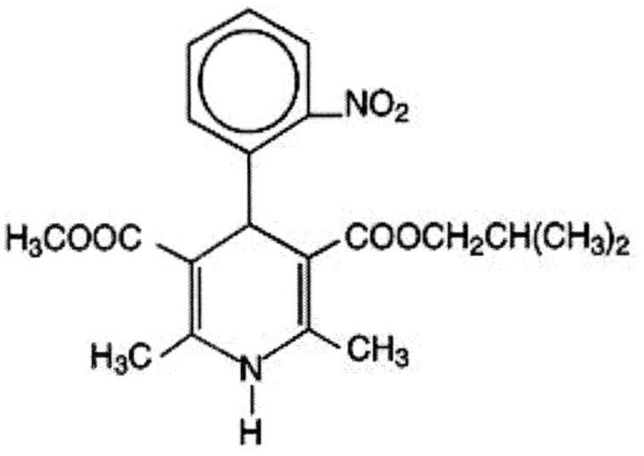

Drug Interactions

Nisoldipine and Atenolol

Potential interactions between nisoldipine and atenolol can occur.

Nisoldipine and Histamine H 2 Receptor Antagonist

A 30 to 45% increase in AUC and C max of nisoldipine was observed with concomitant administration of cimetidine 400 mg twice daily. Ranitidine 150 mg twice daily did not interact significantly with nisoldipine (AUC was decreased by 15-20%). No pharmacodynamic effects of either histamine H 2 receptor antagonist were observed.

ISRADIPINE

Brief Compound Description

Isradipine is a dihydropyridine calcium channel blocker. The structural formula of isradipine is:

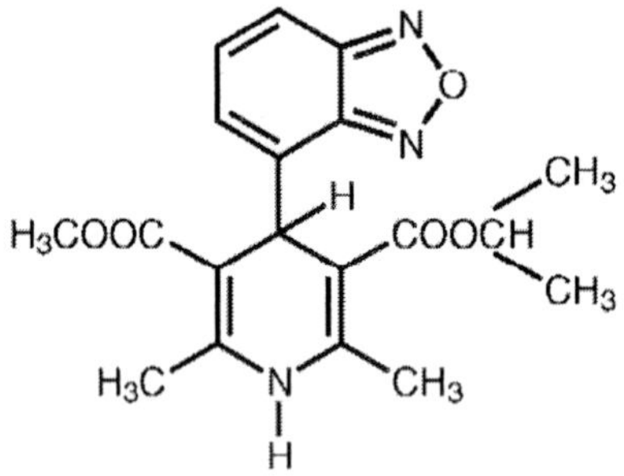

$C_{19}H_{21}N_3O_5$ Mol. wt. 371.39

Drug Interactions

Isradipine and Nitroglycerin

Immediate-release isradipine has been safely coadministered with nitroglycerin.

Isradipine and Hydrochlorothiazide

Concomitant administration of isradipine and hydrochlorothiazide does not result in altered pharmacokinetics of either drug.

Isradipine and Propranolol

Co-administration of propranolol had a small effect on the rate but no effect on the extent of isradipine bioavailability. Significant increases in AUC (27%) and C max (58%) and decreases in t max (23%) of propranolol were noted in this study.

Isradipine and Digoxin

The concomitant administration of isradipine and digoxin in a single-dose pharmacokinetic study did not affect renal, non-renal and total body clearance of digoxin.

LACIDIPINE

Brief Compound Description

Lacidipine is a long acting 2, 4-dihydropyridine calcium channel antagonist, C26H33NO6. The structural formula is the following:

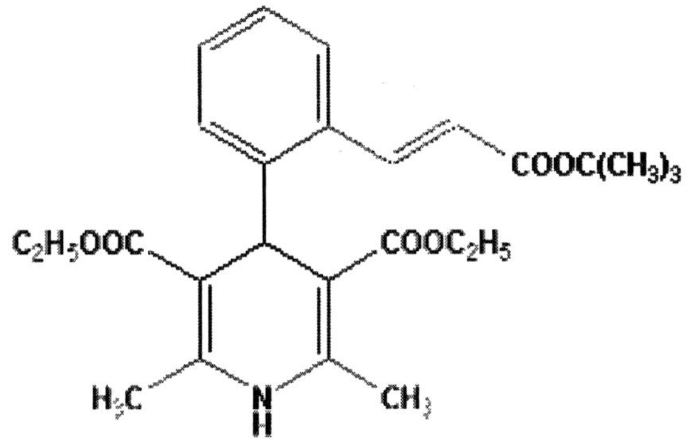

Mechanism of Action

Lacidipine is an orally administered calcium channel blocker of the dihydropyridine class, which shows selectivity for vascular smooth muscle over cardiac tissue and has a long duration of action.

Drug Interactions

Lacidipine and Statins

Lacidipine increased the maximum concentration of simvastatin (Cmax) by approximately 70% and the area under the plasma concentration-time curve AUC (0,24 h) by approximately 35% but coadministration of lacidipine is unlikely to be of clinical relevance [1].

Lacidipine and Propranolol

Propranolol significantly decreased the maximum plasma concentration (Cmax) and area under the plasma concentration-time curve (AUC) of lacidipine (by 38% and 42%, respectively) whereas lacidipine significantly increased the Cmax and AUC of propranolol (by 35% and 26%, respectively). Hence, a modest pharmacokinetic and pharmacodynamic interaction is evident and should be evaluated further in patients with hypertension [2].

References

[1] Ziviani L, Da Ros L, Squassante L, Milleri S, Cugola M, Iavarone LE The effects of lacidipine on the steady/state plasma concentrations of simvastatin in healthy subjects. *Br J Clin Pharmacol.* 2001 Feb;51(2):147-52.

[2] Hall ST, Harding SM, Hassani H, Keene ON, Pellegatti M The pharmacokinetic and pharmacodynamic interaction between lacidipine and propranolol in healthy volunteers. *J Cardiovasc Pharmacol.* 1991;18 Suppl 11:S13-7.

LERCANIDIPINE

Brief Compound Description

Lercanidipine is a dihydropyridine calcium-channel blocker. The structural formula is:

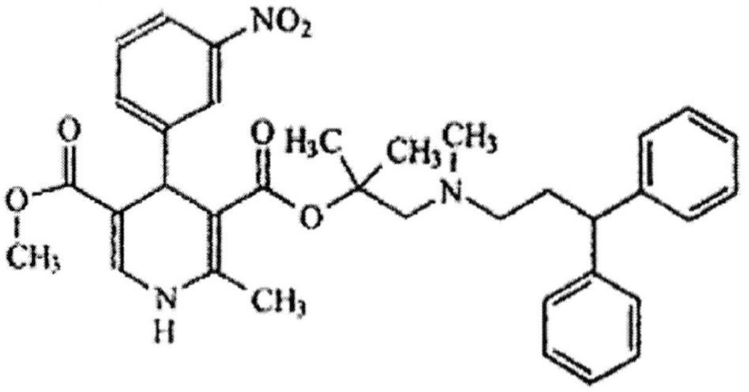

Mechanism of Action

Lercanidipine is a vasoselective dihydropyridine calcium channel antagonist that causes systemic vasodilation by blocking the influx of calcium ions through L-type calcium channels in cell membranes. It is a highly lipophilic drug that exhibits a slower onset and longer duration of action than other calcium channel antagonists

Drug Interactions

The cytochrome P450 (CYP) isoform CYP3A4 and the P-glycoprotein (P-gp), respectively, will have a high impact for both pharmacokinetic processes, as lercanidipine is a substrate of CYP3A4. If inducers or inhibitors of CYP3A4 are concomitantly administered with lercanidipine pharmacokinetic interactions could be expected to a variable extent [1].

References

[1] Klotz U Interaction potential of lercanidipine, a new vasoselective dihydropyridine calcium antagonist. *Arzneimittelforschung.* 2002;52(3):155-61

NICARDIPINE

Brief Compound Description

Nicardipine hydrochloride is a dihydropyridine structure with the IUPAC (International Union of Pure and Applied Chemistry) chemical name 2-(benzyl-methyl amino)ethyl methyl

1,4-dihydro-2,6-dimethyl-4-(m-nitrophenyl)-3,5- pyridinedicarboxylate monohydrochloride, and it has the following structural formula:

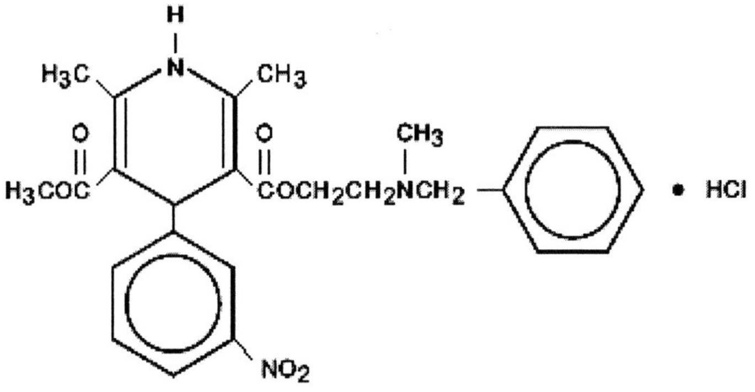

$C_{26}H_{29}N_3O_6 \bullet HCl$

Drug Interactions

Nicardipine and Beta-Blockers

No clinicall significant interactions when adrenergic beta-receptor blockers have been frequently administered concomitantly with nicardipine

Nicardipine and Cimetidine

Cimetidine increases nicardipine plasma levels. Patients receiving the two drugs concomitantly should be carefully monitored.

Nicardipine and Digoxin

Nicardipine usually does ot alter the plasma levels of digoxin, however, serum digoxin levels should be evaluated after concomitant therapy withnicardipine hydrochloride is initiated.

MANIDIPINE

Brief Compound Description

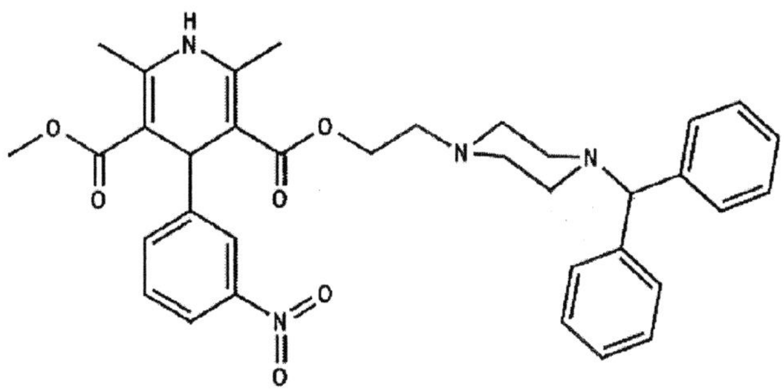

Mechanism of Action

Manidipine is a dihydropyridine calcium antagonist, which causes systemic vasodilation by inhibiting the voltage-dependent calcium inward currents in smooth muscle cells

BEPRIDIL

Brief Compound Description

Bepridil 1-Isobutoxy-2-pyrrolidino-3-(N-benzylanilino)propane. HCl is a non-selective Ca^{2+} channel blocker. Stimulates the binding of 1,4-dihydropyridine-based drugs to Ca^{2+} channels, it inhibits Na^{+}/Ca^{2+} exchange. Th e structural formula is the following:

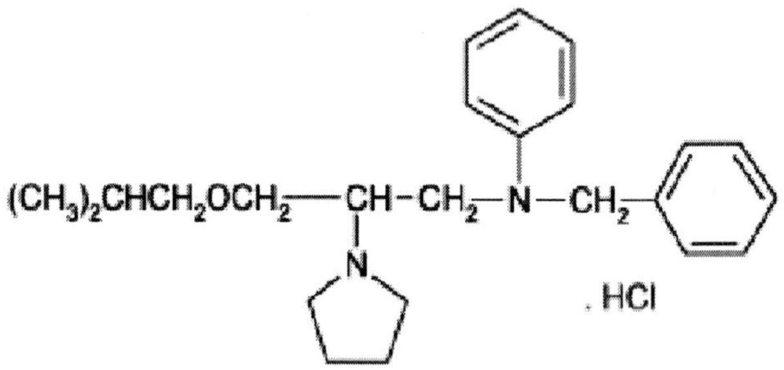

$(CH_3)_2CHCH_2OCH_2$—CH-CH_2—N—CH_2

N

. HCl

Drug Interactions

Bepridil and Nitrates

No drug interactions between bepridil and nitrates

Bepridil and Beta-Blockers

The concomitant use of bepridil and beta-blocking agents has been well tolerated in patients with stable angina.

Bepridil and Digoxin

Bepridil had no effect or was associated with modest increases, about 30% in steady-state digoxin concentrations.

Bepridil and Oral Hypoglycemics

No drug interactions between bepridil and oral hypoglycemic agents have been reported.

ACE INHIBITORS

Mechanism of Action

The mechanism of action of ACE inhibitors has not yet been fully elucidated. Their beneficial effects in hypertension and heart failure appear to result primarily from suppression of the renin-angiotensin-aldosterone system. ACE inhibitors prevent the conversion of angiotensin I to angiotensin II by inhibition of ACE, a peptidyldipeptide carboxy hydrolase. ACE is identical to "bradykininase", and ACE inhibitors may also interfere with the degradation of the vasodepressor peptide, bradykinin. Increased concentrations of bradykinin or prostaglandin E 2 may also have a role in the therapeutic effect of ACE inhibitors. Inhibition of ACE results in decreased plasma angiotensin II and increased plasma renin activity (PRA), the latter resulting from loss of negative feedback on renin release caused by reduction in angiotensin II. The reduction of angiotensin II leads to decreased aldosterone secretion, and, as a result, small increases in serum potassium may occur along with sodium and fluid loss.

The antihypertensive effects persist for a longer period of time than does demonstrable inhibition of circulating ACE. It is not known whether the ACE present in vascular endothelium is inhibited longer than the ACE in circulating blood.

Main of the possible drug-drug interactions between ACE-inhbitors and other components used in patients with metabolic syndrome are summarized in Table 1. The mechanisms and some of these potential interactions are discussed in detail below.

Table 1. Possible drug-drug interactions with ACE-inhibitors in metabolic syndrome

YES	Mechanism and effect	NO
Spironolactone Triamterene Amiloride	+ hyperkalemia	Beta blockers Nitrates Ca-blocking agents
NASIDs	- renal function	Hydralazine Digoxin

HIGHLIGHTS

ACE-inhibitors, with no great differences among each drug, can be safely co-administred with most of other drugs used for the treatment of patients with metabolic syndrome. However a potential interaction of ACE-inhibitors with potassium-sparing diuretics could occur.

ENALAPRIL

Brief Compound Description

Enalapril maleate is chemically described as (S)-1-[N-[1-(ethoxycarbonyl)-3-phenylpropyl]-L-alanyl]-L-proline, (Z)-2-butenedioate salt (1:1). Its empirical formula is C20H28N2O5·C4H404, and its structural formula is

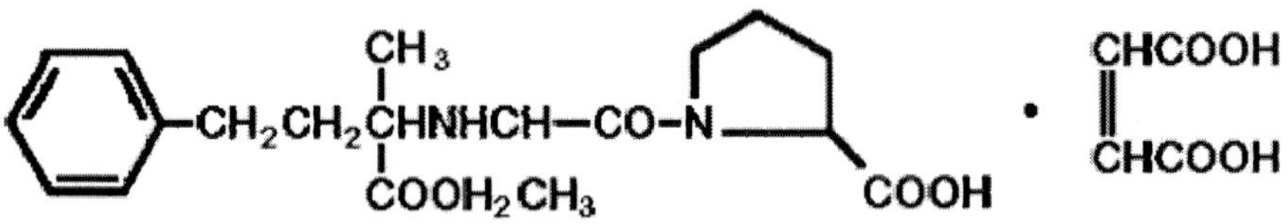

CH_3

$-CH_2CH_2CHNHCH-CO-N$

$COOH_2CH_3$ COOH • CHCOOH ‖ CHCOOH

Drug Interactions

Enalapril and Diuretics

An excessive reduction of blood pressure when diuretics are co- therapy with enalapril. The possibility of hypotensive effects with enalapril can be minimized by either discontinuing the diuretic or increasing the salt intake prior to initiation of treatment with enalapril. The antihypertensive effect of Enalapril is also augmented by diuretics that cause renin release.

Enalapril and Potassium-sparing Diuretics

Enalapril attenuates potassium loss caused by thiazide-type diuretics. Potassium-sparing diuretics (e.g., spironolactone, triamterene, or amiloride), potassium supplements, or potassium-containing salt-substitutes may lead to significant increases in serum potassium. Therefore, if concomitant use of these agents is indicated because of demonstrated hypokalemia, they should be used with caution and with frequent monitoring of serum potassium. Potassium sparing agents should generally not be used in patients with heart failure receiving Enalapril.

Enalapril and Other Cardiovascular Agents

Enalapril has been used concomitantly with beta adrenergic-blocking agents, nitrates, calcium-blocking agents, hydralazine, and digoxin without evidence of clinically significant adverse interactions.

Enalapril and Non-Steroidal Anti-Inflammatory Medicines

In patients with compromised renal function treated with non-steroidal anti-inflammatory drugs, the coadministration of Enalapril may result in a further deterioration of renal function. These effects are usually reversible.

FOSINOPRIL

Brief Compound Description

Fosinopril sodium's chemical name is L-proline, 4-cyclohexyl-1-[[[2-methyl-1-(1-oxopropoxy)- propoxy]-(4 phenylbutyl)- phosphinyl]acetyl]-, sodium salt, trans -; its structural formula is:

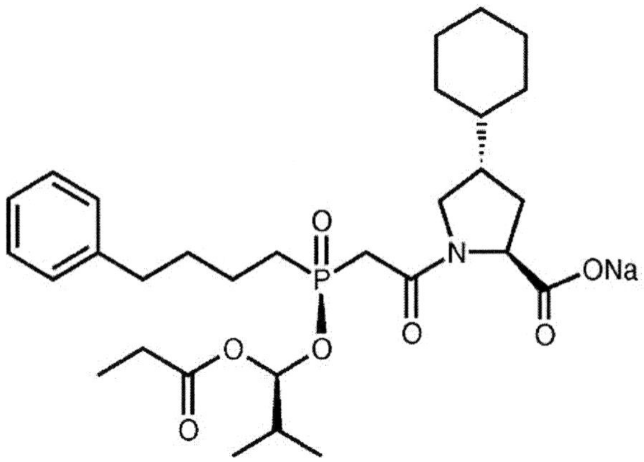

Drug Interactions

Fosinopril and Potassium Supplements and Potassium-Sparing Diuretics

Potassium-sparing diuretics (spironolactone, amiloride, triamterene, and others) or potassium supplements can increase the risk of hyperkalemia. If concomitant use of such agents is indicated, they should be given with caution, and the patients serum potassium should be monitored frequently.

Fosinopril and Warfarin

Interaction studies with warfarin have failed to identify any clinically important effects of fosinopril on the serum concentration or clinical effects of the anticoagulant.

CAPTOPRIL

Brief Compound Description

Captopril is a specific competitive inhibitor of angiotensin I-converting enzyme (ACE), the enzyme responsible for the conversion of angiotensin I to angiotensin II. Captopril is designated chemically as 1-[2S)-3-mercapto-2-methylpropionyl]-L-proline. The structural formula is:

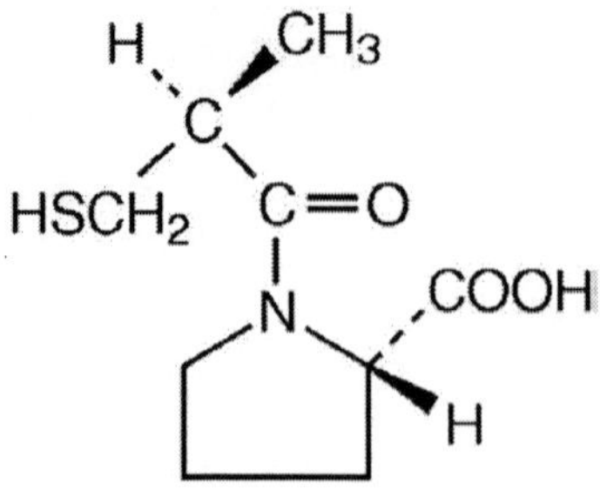

$C_9H_{15}NO_3S$

Drug Interactions

Captopril and Diuretics

Patients on diuretics and especially those in whom diuretic therapy was recently instituted, may occasionally experience a precipitous reduction of blood pressure usually within the first hour after receiving the initial dose of captopril. For example, thiazides may activate the renin-angiotensin-aldosterone system

Captopril and Potassium-sparing Diuretics

Since captopril decreases aldosterone production, elevation of serum potassium may occur. Potassium-sparing diuretics such as spironolactone, triamterene, or amiloride, or potassium supplements should be given only for documented hypokalemia, and then with caution, since they may lead to a significant increase of serum potassium. Salt substitutes containing potassium should also be used with caution.

Captopril and Loop Diuretics

Furosemide administered concurrently with captopril does not alter the pharmacokinetics of captopril in renally impaired hypertensive patients.

Captopril and Agents Having Vasodilator Activity

Data on the effect of concomitant use of other vasodilators in patients receiving captopril for heart failure are not available; therefore, nitroglycerin or other nitrates or other drugs having vasodilator activity should, if possible, be discontinued before starting captopril. If resumed during captopril therapy, such agents should be administered cautiously, and perhaps at lower dosage.

Captopril and Beta-blockers

Beta-adrenergic blocking drugs add some further antihypertensive effect to captopril, but the overall response is less than additive.

Captopril and Inhibitors of Endogenous Prostaglandin Synthesis

It has been reported that indomethacin may reduce the antihypertensive effect of captopril, especially in cases of low renin hypertension. Other nonsteroidal anti-inflammatory agents (e.g., aspirin) may also have this effect.

Captopril and Digoxin

In a study of young healthy male subjects no evidence of a direct pharmacokinetic captopril-digoxin interaction could be found.

Captopril and Allopurinol

In a study of healthy male volunteers no significant pharmacokinetic interaction occurred when captopril and allopurinol were administered concomitantly for 6 days.

PERINDOPRIL

Brief Compound Description

Perindopril erbumine is chemically described as (2S,3(infinity)S,7(infinity)S)-1-[S)-N-[S)-1-Carboxybutyl]alanyl]hexahydro-2-indolinecarboxylic acid, 1-ethyl ester, compound with tert-butylamine (1:1). Its molecular formula is C 19 H 32 N 2 O 5 C 4 H 11 N. Its structural formula is

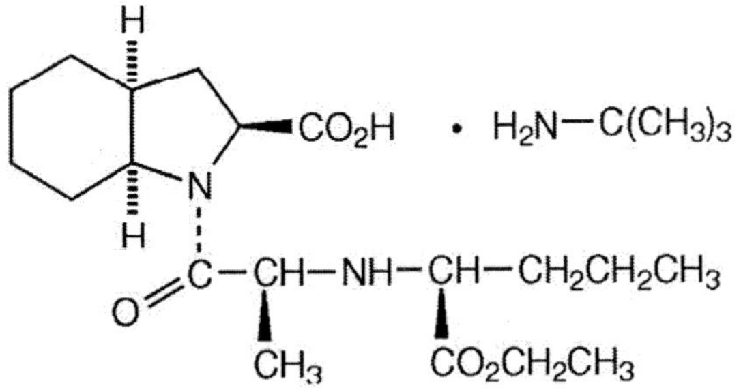

Drug Interactions

Perindopril and Diuretics

Patients on diuretics and especially those started recently, may occasionally experience an excessive reduction of blood pressure after initiation of Perindopril therapy.

Perindopril and Potassium-sparing Diuretics

Perindopril may increase serum potassium because of its potential to decrease aldosterone production. Use of potassium-sparing diuretics (spironolactone, amiloride, triamterene and others), potassium supplements or other drugs capable of increasing serum potassium (heparin) can increase the risk of hyperkalemia. Therefore, if concomitant use of such agents is indicated, they should be given with caution and the patient's serum potassium should be monitored frequently.

Perindopril and Digoxin

A controlled pharmacokinetic study has shown no effect on plasma digoxin concentrations when coadministered with Perindopril,, but an effect of digoxin on the plasma concentration of perindopril/perindoprilat has not been excluded.

LISINOPRIL

Brief Compound Description

Lisinopril is an oral long-acting angiotensin converting enzyme inhibitor. Lisinopril, a synthetic peptide derivative, is chemically described as (S)-1-[N^2 -(1-carboxy-3-phenylpropyl)-L-lysyl]-L-proline dihydrate. Its empirical formula is $C_{21}H_{31}N_3O_5 \cdot 2H_2O$ and its structural formula is:

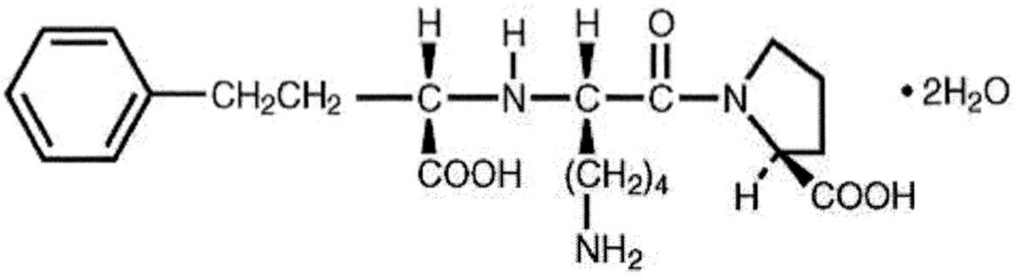

Drug Interactions

Lisinopril and Diuretics

As for other ACE-inhibitors an excessive reduction of blood pressure after initiation of therapy with Lisinopril when diuretics are concomitant can occur. Studies with ACE inhibitors in combination with diuretics indicate that the dose of the ACE inhibitor can be reduced when it is given with a diuretic.

Lisinopril and Agents Increasing Serum Potassium

Lisinopril attenuates potassium loss caused by thiazide-type diuretics. Use of Lisinopril with potassium-sparing diuretics (e.g., spironolactone, triamterene or amiloride), potassium supplements, or potassium-containing salt substitutes may lead to significant increases in serum potassium. Therefore, if concomitant use of these agents is indicated because of demonstrated hypokalemia, they should be used with caution and with frequent monitoring of serum potassium.

Lisinopril and Indomethacin

A study in hypertensive patients showed that when Lisinopril was given concomitantly with indomethacin, the use of indomethacin was associated with a reduced hypotensive effect, although the difference between the two regimens was not significant.

Lisinopril and Other Agents

Lisinopril has been used concomitantly with nitrates and/or digoxin without evidence of clinically significant adverse interactions. No clinically important pharmacokinetic interactions occurred when Lisinopril was used concomitantly with propranolol or hydrochlorothiazide.

QUINAPRIL

Brief Compound Description

Quinapril hydrochloride is chemically described as [3S-[2[R*(R*], 3R*]]-2-[2-[[1-(ethoxycarbonyl)-3-phenylpropyl]amino]-1-oxopropyl]-1,2,3,4-tetrahydro-3-isoquinolinecarboxylic acid, monohydrochloride. Its empirical formula is $C_{25}H_{30}N_{2}O_{5}$ ·HCl and its structural formula is:

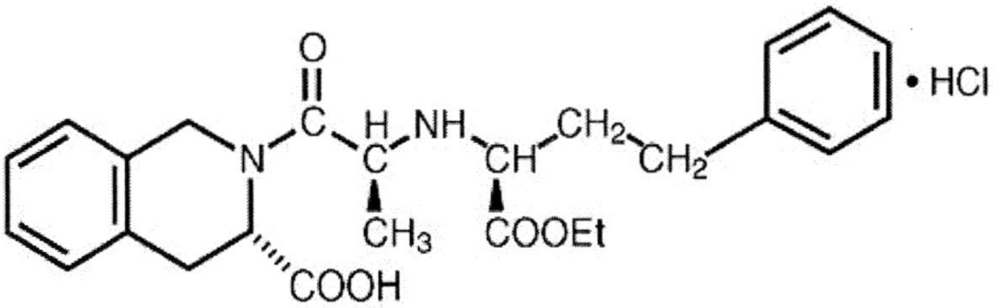

M.W.=474.98

Drug Interactions

Quinapril and Diuretics

As with other ACE inhibitors, patients on diuretics, especially those on recently instituted diuretic therapy, may occasionally experience an excessive reduction of blood pressure after initiation of therapy with Quininapril.

Quinapril and Agents Increasing Serum Potassium

Quinapril can attenuate potassium loss caused by thiazide diuretics and increase serum potassium when used alone. If concomitant therapy of Quininapril with potassium-sparing diuretics (eg, spironolactone, triamterene, or amiloride), potassium supplements, or potassium-containing salt substitutes is indicated, they should be used with caution along with appropriate monitoring of serum potassium

No Drug interactions between *Quinapril and propranolol, warfarin, digoxin, atorvastatin, hydrochlothiazide or cimetidine* were observed.

RAMIPRIL

Brief Compound Description

Ramipril is a 2-aza-bicyclo [3.3.0]-octane-3-carboxylic acid derivative. Ramipril's chemical name is (2S,3aS,6aS)-1[S)-N-[S)-l-Carboxy-3-phenylpropyl]-alanyl]octahydrocyclopenta[b]pyrrole-2-carboxylic acid, 1-ethyl ester; its structural formula is:

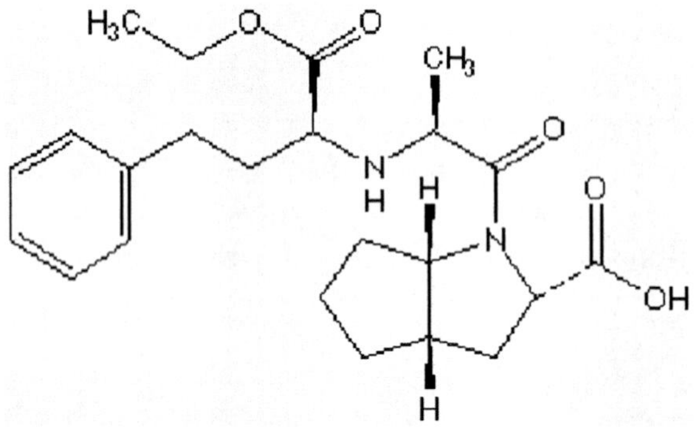

Drug Interactions

Ramipril and Diuretics

Patients on diuretics, especially those in whom diuretic therapy was recently instituted, may occasionally experience an excessive reduction of blood pressure after initiation of therapy with ramipril.

Ramipril and Potassium Sparing Diuretics

Ramipril can attenuate potassium loss caused by thiazide diuretics. Potassium sparing diuretics (spironolactone, amiloride, triamterene and others), potassium supplements can increase the risk of hyperkalaemia. Therefore, if concomitant use of such agents is indicated, they should be given with caution, and the patient's serum potassium should be monitored frequently.

Ramipril and NSAIDS

As with other ACE inhibitors, the antihypertensive effects of ramipril may be decreased in patients taking non-steroidal anti-inflammatory drugs (eg. acetylsalicylic acid, phenylbutazone, indomethacin).

Ramipril and Antidiabetic Agents

The possibility of an increased blood sugar reduction must be considered in patients treated concurrently with ramipril and antidiabetic agents such as insulin and sulphonylurea derivatives.

ANGIOTENSIN II RECEPTOR ANTAGONISTS (AIIRAS) (SARTANS)

Angiotensin II is a potent vasoconstrictor, the primary vasoactive hormone of the renin-angiotensin system and an important component in the pathophysiology of hypertension. It also stimulates aldosterone secretion by the adrenal cortex. Angiotensin II receptor antagonists (AIIRAS) block the vasoconstrictor and aldosterone-secreting effects of angiotensin II by selectively blocking the binding of angiotensin II to the AT 1 receptor found in many tissues, (e.g., vascular smooth muscle, adrenal gland). There is also an AT 2 receptor found in many tissues but it is not known to be associated with cardiovascular homeostasis.

General Drug Interactions

All sartans except eprosartan have at least some affinity for CYP2C9, but only losartan has an affinity for CYP2C19. Losartan and irbesartan have modest affinity for CYP1A2 and CYP3A4. This would suggest that the theoretical potential for drug interactions is likely to be quite low, with the possible exceptions of losartan and irbesartan for CYP2C9 [1]. The difference on sartans metabolism by cytochrome P450 are summarized in table 1

Table 1. AIIRAs biotrasformation in relation to cytochrome P450

P450	No P450
Losartan	Valsartan
Irbersartan	Candesartan
	Telimisartan
	Eprosartan
	Olmesartan

HIGHLIGHTS

Sartans, with no great differences among each drug, can be safely co-administred with the drugs used for the treatment of patients with metabolic syndrome. However, since valsartan, candesartan, telmisartan, eprosartan, olmesartan are not significantly metabolized by the cytochrome P450 system and at therapeutic concentrations have no effects on P450 enzymes, interactions with drugs that inhibit or are metabolized by those enzymes would not be expected

References

[1] Taavitsainen P, Kiukaanniemi K, Pelkonen O. In vitro inhibition screening of human hepatic P450 enzymes by five angiotensin-II receptor antagonists. *Eur J Clin Pharmacol.* 2000 May;56(2):135-40.

LOSARTAN

Brief Compound Description

Losartan is an angiotensin II receptor (type AT_1) antagonist. Losartan potassium, a non-peptide molecule, is chemically described as 2-butyl-4-chloro-1-[p -(o-1 H -tetrazol-5-ylphenyl)benzyl]imidazole-5-methanol monopotassium salt. Its empirical formula is $C_{22}H_{22}ClKN_6O$, and its structural formula is:

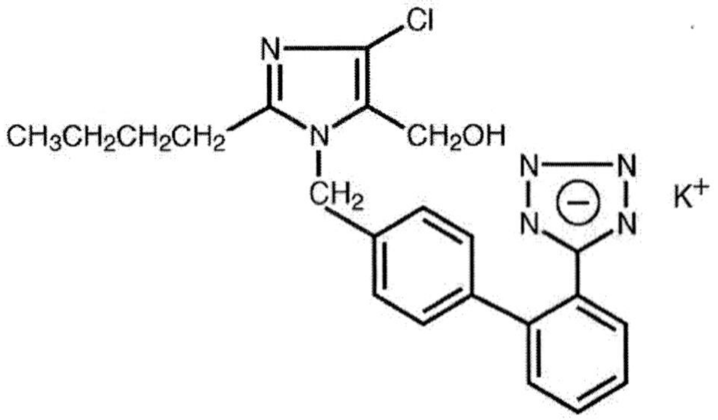

Drug Interactions

Losartan is an orally active agent that undergoes substantial first-pass metabolism by cytochrome P450 enzymes. It is converted, in part, to an active carboxylic acid metabolite that is responsible for most of the angiotensin II receptor antagonism that follows losartan treatment. Losartan metabolites have been identified in human plasma and urine. In addition to the active carboxylic acid metabolite, several inactive metabolites are formed. In vitro studies indicate that cytochrome P450 2C9 and 3A4 are involved in the biotransformation of losartan to its metabolites.

Losartan and Warfarin

Losartan, administered for 12 days, did not affect the pharmacokinetics or pharmacodynamics of a single dose of warfarin.

Losartan and Digoxin

Losartan did not affect the pharmacokinetics of oral or intravenous digoxin.

Losartan and Hydrochlorothiazide

There is no pharmacokinetic interaction between losartan and hydrochlorothiazide.

Losartan and Orlistat

No interactions between Losartan and Orlistat were observed [1].

Losartan and Nitroglycerin

The venodilation caused by nitroglycerin was decreased by angiotensin II, and this effect was attenuated by pretreatment with losartan [2].

Losartan and NSAIDs

NSAIDs are known to attenuate the effects of some antihypertensive medications. Concurrent treatment with indomethacin similarly attenuates the 24-hour antihypertensive response to losartan [3]. Although NSAIDs such as indomethacin clearly affect blood pressure, it is not known whether the new class of NSAID agents, cyclooxygenase (COX)-2 inhibitors, will have the same effect

References

[1] Zhi J, Moore R, Kanitra L, Mulligan TE Pharmacokinetic evaluation of the possible interaction between selected concomitant medications and orlistat at steady state in healthy subjects. *J Clin Pharmacol.* 2002 Sep;42(9):1011-9.

[2] Harada K, Sugimoto K, Kawaguchi A, Ohmori M, Fujimura A Effect of angiotensin II on venodilator response to nitroglycerin. *Clin Pharmacol Ther.* 2001 Mar;69(3):130-6

[3] Conlin PR, Moore TJ, Swartz SL, Barr E, Gazdick L, Fletcher C, DeLucca P, Demopoulos L. Effect of indomethacin on blood pressure lowering by captopril and losartan in hypertensive patients. *Hypertension.* 2000 Sep;36(3):461-5.

IRBESARTAN

Brief Compound Description

Irbesartan is an angiotensin II receptor (AT 1 subtype) antagonist. Irbesartan is a non-peptide compound, chemically described as a 2-butyl-3-[p -(o -1 H -tetrazol-5-ylphenyl)benzyl]-1,3-diazaspiro[4,4]non-1-en-4-one. Its empirical formula is C 25 H 28 N 6 O, and the structural formula:

Drug Interactions

Irbesartan is an angiotensin II receptor antagonist indicated for the treatment of patients with hypertension. Although irbesartan does not require biotransformation for its pharmacological activity, it does undergo metabolism via the cytochrome P450 (CYP) 2C9 isoenzyme and negligible metabolism by the CYP3A4 isoenzyme

Irbesartan and Hydrochlorothiazide, Digoxin, Warfarin, Simvastatin, Tolbutamide and Nifedipine

No significant drug-drug pharmacokinetic (or pharmacodynamic) interactions have been found in interaction studies with hydrochlorothiazide, digoxin, warfarin, simvastatin, tolbutamide and nifedipine [1].

References

[1] Marino MR, Vachharajani NN Drug interactions with irbesartan. Clin Pharmacokinet. 2001;40(8):605-14.

VALSARTAN

Brief Compound Description

Valsartan is a nonpeptide, orally active, and specific angiotensin II antagonist acting on the AT 1 receptor subtype. Valsartan is chemically described as N -(1-oxopentyl)- N -[[2'-(1 H -tetrazol-5-yl) [1,1'-biphenyl]-4-yl]methyl]-L-valine. Its empirical formula is $C_{24}H_{29}N_5O_3$, its molecular weight is 435.5, and its structural formula is

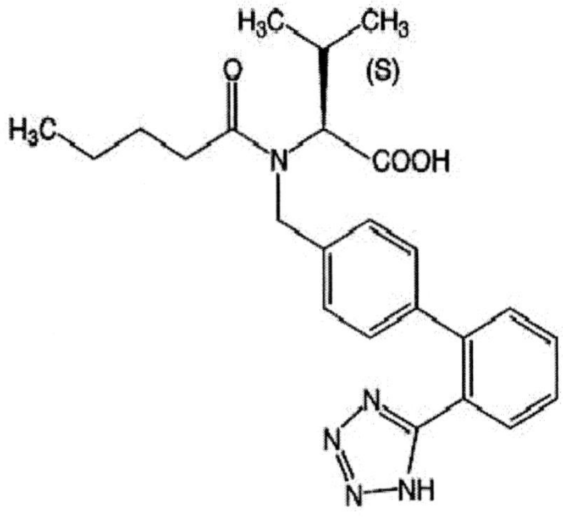

Drug Interactions

The enzymes) responsible for valsartan metabolism have not been identified but do not seem to be CYP 450 isozmes. The inhibitory or induction potential of valsartan on CYP 450 is also unknown.

Valsartan and Amlodipine, Atenolol, Cimetidine, Digoxin, Furosemide, Glyburide, Hydrochlorothiazide, Warfarin or Indomethacin

No clinically significant pharmacokinetic interactions were observed when valsartan was coadministered with amlodipine, atenolol, cimetidine, digoxin, furosemide, glyburide, hydrochlorothiazide, warfarin or indomethacin.

Valsartan and Atenolol

The valsartan-atenolol combination was more antihypertensive than either component, but it did not lower the heart rate more than atenolol alone.

Valsartan and Potassium Sparing Diuretics

As with other drugs that block angiotensin II or its effects, concomitant use of potassium sparing diuretics (e.g., spironolactone, triamterene, amiloride), potassium supplements, or salt substitutes containing potassium may lead to increases in serum potassium and in heart failure patients to increases in serum creatinine.

CANDESARTAN

Brief Compound Description

Candesartan cilexetil, a nonpeptide, is chemically described as. (±)-1-Hydroxyethyl 2-ethoxy-1-[p -(o -1 H -tetrazol-5-ylphenyl)benzyl]-7-benzimidazolecarboxylate, cyclohexyl carbonate (ester). Its empirical formula is $C_{33}H_{34}N_6O_6$, and its structural formula is

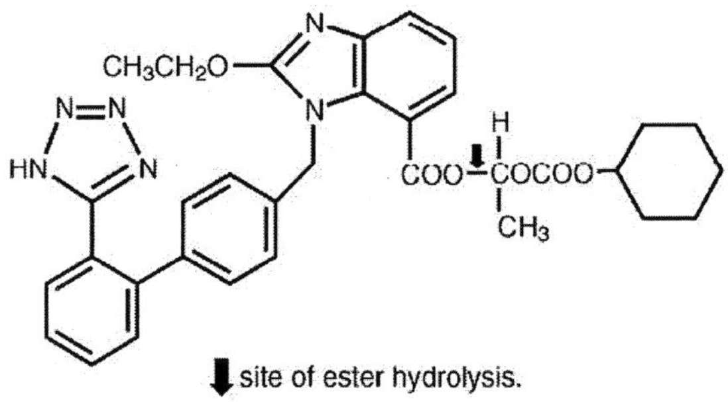

CH_3CH_2O N=N HN N N N H COO COCOO CH_3

site of ester hydrolysis.

Drug Interactions

Since candesartan is not significantly metabolized by the cytochrome P450 system and at therapeutic concentrations has no effects on P450 enzymes, interactions with drugs that inhibit or are metabolized by those enzymes would not be expected.

Candesartan and Glyburide, Nifedipine, Digoxin, Warfarin, Hydrochlorothiazide, and Oral Contraceptives

No significant drug interactions have been reported in studies of candesartan cilexetil given with other drugs such as glyburide, nifedipine, digoxin, warfarin, hydrochlorothiazide, and oral contraceptives in healthy volunteers.

TELMISARTAN

Brief Compound Description

Telmisartan is a nonpeptide angiotensin II receptor (type AT_1) antagonist. Telmisartan is chemically described as 4'-[1,4'-dimethyl-2'-propyl[2,6'-bi-1H-benzimidazol]-1'-yl)methyl]-[1,1'-biphenyl]-2-carboxylic acid. Its empirical formula is $C_{33}H_{30}N_4O_2$, its molecular weight is 514.63, and its structural formula is:

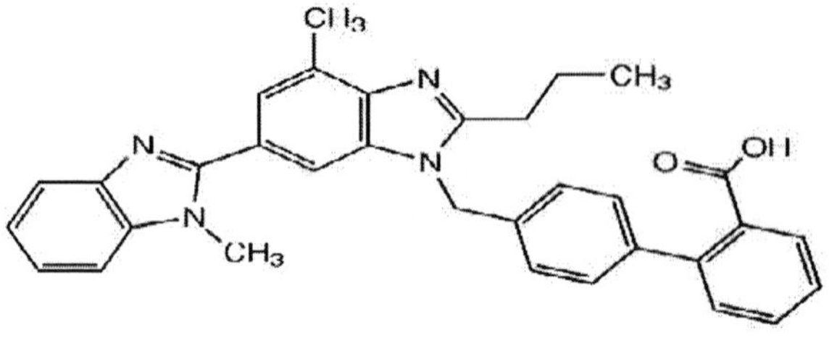

Drug Interactions

Telmisartan is not metabolized by the cytochrome P450 system and had no effects in vitro on cytochrome P450 enzymes, except for some inhibition of CYP2C19. Telmisartan is not expected to interact with drugs that inhibit cytochrome P450 enzymes; it is also not expected to interact with drugs metabolized by cytochrome P450 enzymes, except for possible inhibition of the metabolism of drugs metabolized by CYP2C19.

Telmisartan and Digoxin

When telmisartan was coadministered with digoxin, median increases in digoxin peak plasma concentration (49%) and in trough concentration (20%) were observed. It is, therefore, recommended that digoxin levels be monitored when initiating, adjusting, and discontinuing telmisartan to avoid possible over- or under-digitalization.

Nevertheless, since any symptoms of overdose are related only to steady state and not peak concentrations and due to the fact that there was a lack of effect on serum trough levels of digoxin, it is unlikely that the findings have any clinical relevance. The magnitude of increase in digoxin concentrations is comparable with increases observed with administration of calcium antagonists, carvedilol, ACE inhibitors such as captopril, and antiarrhythmic drugs such as amiodarone, quinidine, and Propafenone. Monitoring of serum digoxin concentrations should be considered when patients first receive telmisartan and in the event of any changes in telmisartan dose [1].

Telmisartan and Warfarin

Telmisartan administered for 10 days slightly decreased the mean warfarin trough plasma concentration; this decrease did not result in a change in International Normalized Ratio (INR).

Telmisartan and Acetaminophen, Amlodipine, Glibenclamide, Simvastatin, Hydrochlorothiazide or Ibuprofen

Coadministration of telmisartan did not result in a clinically significant interaction with acetaminophen, amlodipine, glibenclamide, simvastatin, hydrochlorothiazide or ibuprofen.

References

[1] Stangier J, Su CA, Hendriks MG, van Lier JJ, Sollie FA, Oosterhuis B, Jonkman JH. The effect of telmisartan on the steady-state pharmacokinetics of digoxin in healthy male volunteers. *J Clin Pharmacol.* 2000 Dec;40(12 Pt 1):1373-9.

EPROSARTAN

Brief Compound Description

Eprosartan mesylate is a nonbiphenyl non-tetrazole angiotensin II receptor (AT_1) antagonist. A selective non-peptide molecule, Eprosartan is chemically described as the monomethanesulfonate of (E)-2-butyl-1-(p-carboxybenzyl)-(alpha)-2- thienylmethylimidazole-5-acrylic acid.

Its empirical formula is $C_{23}H_{24}N_2O_4S \cdot CH_4O_3S$ and molecular weight is 520.625. Its structural formula is:

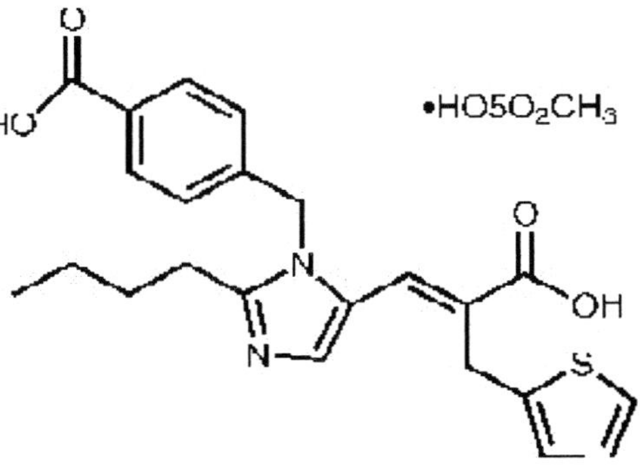

Drug Interactions

Because eprosartan is not metabolized by the cytochrome P450 system, inhibitors of CYP450 enzyme would not be expected to affect its metabolism.

Eprosartan Mesylate and Digoxin and Warfarin and Glyburide

Eprosartan has been shown to have no effect on the pharmacokinetics of digoxin and the pharmacodynamics of warfarin and glyburide.

Eprosartan and Diuretics

Eprosartan has been safely used concomitantly with a thiazide diuretic (hydrochlorothiazide).

Eprosartan and Calcium Channel Blockers

Eprosartan has been safely used concomitantly with sustained-release calcium channel blockers (sustained-release nifedipine) with no clinically significant adverse interactions.

Eprosartan and Potassium-sparing Diuretics

As with other drugs that block angiotensin II or its effects, concomitant use of potassium-sparing diuretics (e.g., spironolactone, triamterene, amiloride), potassium supplements or salt substitutes containing potassium may lead to increases in serum potassium

OLMESARTAN

Brief Compound Description

Olmesartan medoxomil is hydrolyzed to olmesartan during absorption from the gastrointestinal tract. Olmesartan medoxomil is 2,3-dihydroxy-2-butenyl 4-(1-hydroxy-1-methylethyl)-2-propyl-1-[p -(o -1 H -tetrazol-5-ylphenyl)benzyl]imidazole-5-carboxylate, cyclic 2, 3-carbonate.

Its empirical formula is C 29 H 30 N 6 O 6 and its structural formula is:

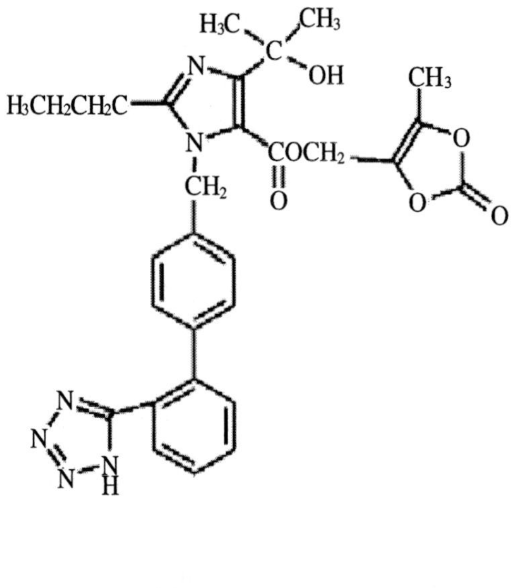

Drug Interactions

Olmesartan is not metabolized by the cytochrome P-450 and has a dual route of elimination, by kidneys and liver. Olmesartan medoxomil has minimal adverse effects with no clinically important drug interactions [1]. Olmesartan medoxomil is not metabolized by the cytochrome P450 system and has no effects on P450 enzymes; thus, interactions with drugs that inhibit, induce or are metabolized by those enzymes are not expected.

No significant drug interactions were reported in studies in which olmesartan medoxomil was co-administered with hydrochlorothiazide, digoxin or warfarin in healthy volunteers. The bioavailability of olmesartan was not significantly altered by the co-administration of antacids.

References

[1] Yoshida K, Kohzuki M. Clinical and experimental aspects of olmesartan medoxomil, a new angiotensin II receptor antagonist.Cardiovasc Drug Rev. 2004 Winter;22(4):285-308

OMAPATRILAT

Omapatrilat is a vasopeptidase inhibitor (VPI) developed for the treatment of hypertension and heart failure. The in vitro effects of omapatrilat, a dual vasopeptidase inhibitor that simultaneously inhibits neutral endopeptidase (NEP) and angiotensin-converting enzyme (ACE).

Drug interactions

Omapatrilat and Furosemide

Daily coadministration of omapatrilat 10 or 25 mg with furosemide 20 mg does not affect the pharmacodynamics offurosemide at steady state [1].

References

[1] Uderman H, Vesterqvist O, Manning J Jr, Ferreira I, Delaney C, Liao WC. Omapatrilat: neurohormonal and pharmacodynamic profile when administered with furosemide. *J Clin Pharmacol.* 2001 Dec;41(12):1291-300

Beta-Blockers

Propranolol

Brief Compound Description

The active ingredient in InnoPran XL is a synthetic beta-adrenergic receptor-blocking agent chemically described as 1-(Isopropylamino)-3-(1-naphthyloxy)-2-propanol hydrochloride. Its structural formula is:

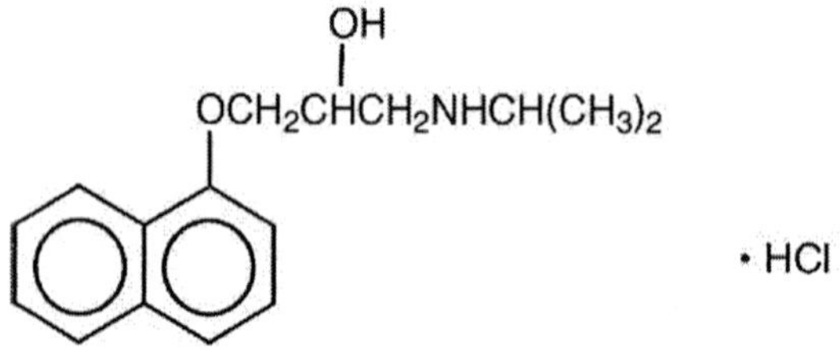

OH

$OCH_2CHCH_2NHCH(CH_3)_2$

· HCl

Mechanism of Action

Propranolol is a nonselective, beta-adrenergic receptor-blocking agent possessing no other autonomic nervous system activity. It specifically competes with beta-adrenergic receptor-stimulating agents for available receptor sites. When access to beta-receptor sites is blocked by propranolol, chronotropic, inotropic, and vasodilator responses to beta-adrenergic stimulation are decreased proportionately. At dosages greater than required for beta blockade, propranolol also exerts a quinidine-like or anesthetic-like membrane action, which affects the cardiac action potential. The significance of the membrane action in the treatment of arrhythmias is uncertain. The mechanism of the antihypertensive effect of propranolol has not been established. Among factors that contribute to the antihypertensive action are: (1) decreased cardiac output, (2) inhibition of renin release by the kidneys, and (3) diminution of tonic sympathetic nerve outflow from vasomotor centers in the brain.

Drug Interactions

Main of the possible drug-drug interactions between propranolol and other components used in patients with metabolic syndrome are summarized in Table 1. The mechanisms and some of these potential interactions are discussed in detail below.

Interactions with Substrates, Inhibitors or Inducers of Cytochrome P-450 Enzymes

Because propranolol's metabolism involves multiple pathways in the cytochrome P-450 system (CYP2D6, 1A2, 2C19), administration of Propranolol with drugs that are metabolized by, or affect the activity (induction or inhibition) of one or more of these pathways may lead to clinically relevant drug interactions.

Substrates or Inhibitors of CYP2D6

Blood levels and/or toxicity of propranolol may be increased by co-administration with substrates or inhibitors of CYP2D6, such as amiodarone, cimetidine and quinidine. No interactions were observed with either ranitidine or lansoprazole.

Substrates or Inhibitors of CYP1A2

Blood levels and/or toxicity of propranolol may be increased by co-administration with substrates or inhibitors of CYP1A2, such as cimetidine.

Substrates or Inhibitors of CYP2C19

Blood levels and/or toxicity of propranolol may be increased by co-administration of propranolol with substrates or inhibitors of CYP2C19, such as cimetidine and tolbutamide. No interaction was observed with omeprazole.

Table 1. Possible drug-drug interactions with propranolol in metabolic syndrome

YES	Mechanism and effect	NO	Potential	Effect
Amiodarone Propafenone	↑ increased concentration of Amiodarone and Propafenone	Diltiazem Fluvastatin	Lovastatin Pravastatin ↓	↓ decreased concentration of statins
	⇑ increased concentration of propranolol	Omeprazole		
Lidocaine Quinidine	⇑ increased concentration of propranolol			
Nisoldipine Nicardipine Nifedipine Verapamil	⇓ decreased absorption and concentration of propranolol			
	⇑ increased concentration of propranolol			
Cholestiramine	⇒ increased prothrombin time			
Tolbutamide	⇑ increased concentration of propranolol			
Warfarin				
Cimetidine				

Inducers of Hepatic Drug Metabolism

Blood levels of propranolol may be decreased by co-administration with inducers such as ethanol. Cigarette smoking also induces hepatic metabolism and has been shown to increase up to 100% the clearance of propranolol, resulting in decreased plasma concentrations.

Propranolol and Antiarrhythmics

The AUC of Propafenone is increased by more than 200% by co-administration of propranolol. The metabolism of propranolol is reduced by co-administration of quinidine, leading to a two-three fold increase in blood concentrations and greater degrees of clinical beta-blockade. The metabolism of lidocaine is inhibited by co-administration of propranolol, resulting in a 25% increase in lidocaine concentrations.

Propranolol and Calcium Channel Blockers

The mean C max and AUC of propranolol are increased respectively, by 50% and 30% by co-administration of nisoldipine and by 80% and 47%, by co-administration of nicardipine. The mean C max and AUC of nifedipine are increased by 64% and 79%, respectively, by co-administration of propranolol. Propranolol does not affect the pharmacokinetics of verapamil and norverapamil. Diltiazem has been reported to displace propranolol-free fractions significantly. Calcium antagonists can produce more severe cardiac depression in the presence of propranolol because the normal sympathetic compensation is blocked, which is unlikely to be a problem in patients with good cardiac function [1].

Propranolol and Lipid Lowering Drugs

Co-administration of cholestiramine or colestipol with propranolol resulted in up to 50% decrease in propranolol concentrations. Co-administration of propranolol with lovastatin or pravastatin decreased 20% to 25% the AUC of both, but did not alter their pharmacodynamics. Propranolol did not have an effect on the pharmacokinetics of fluvastatin.

Propranolol and Warfarin

Concomitant administration of propranolol and warfarin has been shown to increase warfarin bioavailability and increase prothrombin time.

Carvedilol

Brief Compound Description

Carvedilol is a nonselective β-adrenergic blocking agent with α1-blocking activity. It is ±-1-(Carbazol-4-yloxy)-3-[[2-(o-methoxyphenoxy)ethyl]amino]-2-propanol. The structural formula is:

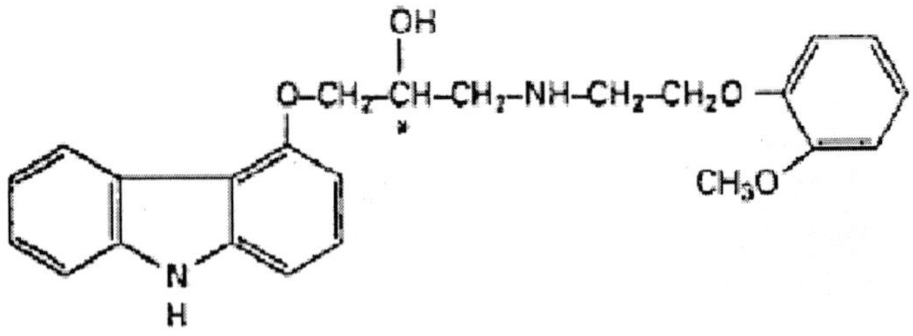

Drug Interactions

Carvedilol and Inhibitors of CYP2D6

Interactions of carvedilol with strong inhibitors of CYP2D6 such as quinidine, and propafen-one have not been studied, but these drugs would be expected to increse blood levels of the R(+) enantiomer of carvedilol.

Carvedilol and Clonidine

Concomitant administration of clonidine With agents with b-blocking properties may potentiate blood-pressure-end heart-rate-lowering effects. When concomitant treatment with agents with b-blocking properties end clonidine is to be terminated, the b-blocking agent should be discontinued first. Clonidine therapy can then be discontinued several days later by gradually decreasing the dosage.

Carvedilol and Digoxin

Digoxin concentrations are increased by about 15% when digoxin and carvedilol are administered concomitantly. Both digoxin and carvedilol slow AV conduction.

Carvedilol and Inducers and Inhibitors of Hepatic Metabolism

Cimetidine increased AUC by about 30% but caused no change in C_{max}.

Carvedilol and Calcium Channel Blockers

Isolated cases of conduction disturbance (rarely with hemodynamic compromise) have been observed when carvedilol is co-administered with diltiazem.

Carvedilol and Oral Hypoglycemics

Agents with b-blocking properties may enhance the blood-sugar-reducing effect of insulin and oral hypoglycemics.

Metoprolol

Brief Compound Description

Metoprolol succinate, is a beta 1 -selective (cardioselective) adrenoceptor blocking agent, for oral administration, available as extended release tablets. Its chemical name is (±)1-

(isopropylamino)-3-[p-(2-methoxyethyl) phenoxy]-2-propanol succinate (2:1) (salt). Its structural formula is:

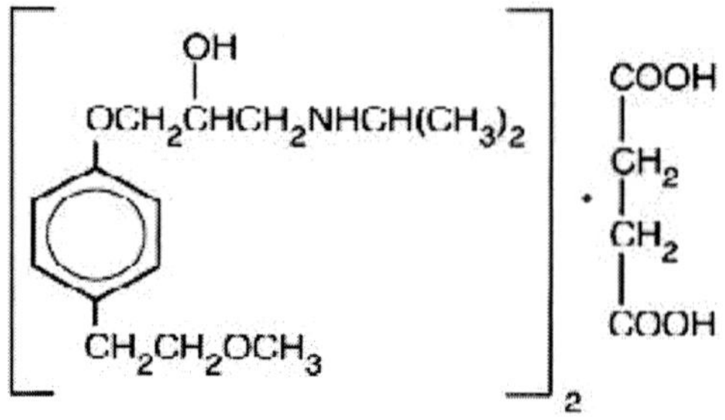

Drug Interactions

Metoprolol is metabolized predominantly by CYP2D6, an enzyme that is absent in about 8% of Caucasians (poor metabolizers) and about 2% of most other populations. CYP2D6 can be inhibited by a number of drugs. Concomitant use of inhibiting drugs in poor metabolizers will increase blood levels of metoprolol several-fold, decreasing metoprolol's cardioselectivity

Metoprolol and Quinidine and Propafenone

Drugs that inhibit CYP2D6 such as quinidine and propafenone are likely to increase metoprolol concentration. In healthy subjects with CYP2D6 extensive metabolizer phenotype, coadministration of quinidine 100 mg and immediate release metoprolol 200 mg tripled the concentration of S-metoprolol and doubled the metoprolol elimination half-life. Coadministration of Propafenone 150 mg t.i.d. with immediate release metoprolol 50 mg t.i.d. resulted in two- to five-fold increases in the steady-state concentration of metoprolol. These increases in plasma concentration would decrease the cardioselectivity of metoprolol.

Metoprolol and Clonidine

Beta-blockers may exacerbate the rebound hypertension which can follow the withdrawal of clonidine. If the two drugs are coadministered, the beta blocker should be withdrawn several days before the gradual withdrawal of clonidine. If replacing clonidine by beta-blocker therapy, the introduction of beta-blockers should be delayed for several days after clonidine administration has stopped.

Atenolol

Brief Compound Description

Atenolol, a synthetic, beta1-selective (cardioselective) adrenoreceptor blocking agent, may be chemically described as benzeneacetamide, 4 -[2'-hydroxy-3'-[1- methylethyl) amino] propoxy]-. The structural formula is:

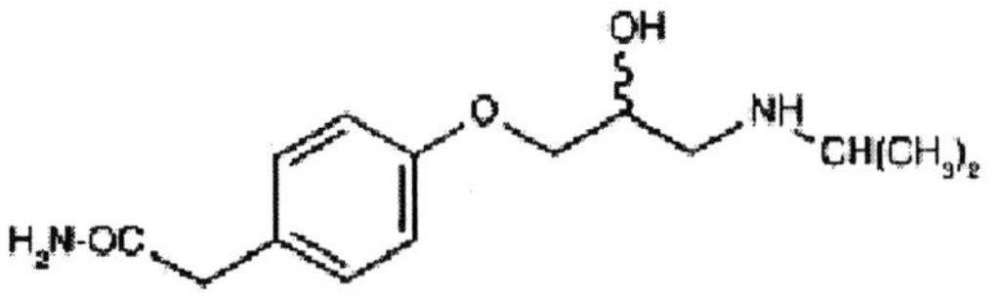

Drug Interactions

Atenolol and Alcohol

Atenolol is not affected by alcohol intake.

Atenolol and Amiodarone

Bradycardia, cardiac arrest, and ventricular fibrillation have been reported when atenolol and amiodarome were coadministred.

Atenolol and Calcium Channel Blockers

Concurrent use has resulted in hypotension, bradycardia, conduction defect, and cardiac failure.

Atenolol and NSAIDS

The anti-hypertensive effects of atenolol may become impaired when taken with NSAIDS.

Atenolol and Antacids

Concurrent use of atenolol and antacids showed a drop in the bioavailability of atenolol. Results are variable for other beta blockers.

Atenolol and Thallium Scans

When patients taking atenolol were taken for a 201 thallous chloride scan their was a marked reduction in the quality of the thallium scans.

Bisoprolol

Brief Compound Description

Bisoprolol is indicated for the treatment of hypertension; it is a synthetic beta 1 -selective (cardioselective) adrenoceptor blocking agent (bisoprolol fumarate). Bisoprolol fumarate is chemically described as (±)-1-[4-[[2-(1-methylethoxy)ethoxy]methyl]phenoxy]-3-[1-methyl-ethyl)amino]-2-propanol(E)-2-butenedioate (2:1) (salt). It possesses an asymmetric carbon atom in its structure and is provided as a racemic mixture. The S(-) enantiomer is responsible for most of the beta-blocking activity. Its empirical formula is (C 18 H 31 NO 4) 2 ·C 4 H 4 O 4 and it has a molecular weight of 766.97. Its structural formula is:

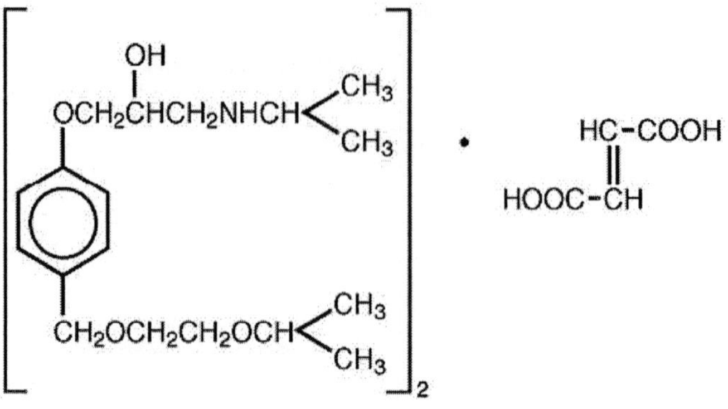

OH

$OCH_2CHCH_2NHCH(CH_3)_2$

$CH_2OCH_2CH_2OCH(CH_3)_2$

2

HC-COOH

HOOC-CH

Drug Interactions

Bisoprolol may potentiate the action of other antihypertensive agents used concomitantly. Bisoprolol should not be combined with other beta-blocking agents. Patients receiving catecholamine-depleting drugs, such as reserpine or guanethidine, should be closely monitored because the added beta-adrenergic blocking action of bisoprolol fumarate may produce excessive reduction of sympathetic activity. In patients receiving concurrent therapy with clonidine, if therapy is to be discontinued, it is suggested that bisoprolol be discontinued for several days before the withdrawal of clonidine.

Bisoprolol should be used with caution when myocardial depressants or inhibitors of AV conduction, such as certain calcium antagonists (particularly of the phenylalkylamine [verapamil] and benzothiazepine [diltiazem] classes), or antiarrhythmic agents, such as disopyramide, are used concurrently

Nebivolol

Brief Compound Description

Nebivolol is a long-acting, cardioselective beta-blocker currently licensed for the treatment of hypertension. It has mild vasodilating properties attributed to its interaction with the L-arginine/nitricoxide pathway, a property not shared by other beta-blockers.Nebivolol is the racemate (dl-nebivolol) of the enantiomers l-nebivolol and d-nebivolol. It is a competitive and highly selective beta-1 receptor antagonist with mild vasodilating properties, possibly due to an interaction with the L-arginine/nitric oxide pathway. Nebivolol is a lipophilic Beta-blocker. The structural formula is:

Drug Interactions

Main of the possible drug-drug interactions between nebivolol and other components used in patients with metabolic syndrome are summarized in Table 1. The mechanisms and some of these potential interactions are discussed in detail below.

Table 1. Potential drug-drug interactions with nebivolol in metabolic syndrome

YES	Mechanism and effect
Verapamil Diltiazem Amiodarone	Increased negative effect on contractility and atrio-ventricular conduction
Digoxin	Increase atrio-ventricular conduction times

Nebivolol and Calcium Antagonists

Caution should be exercised when administering beta-blockers with calcium antagonists of the verapamil or diltiazem type because of their negative effect on contractility and atrio-ventricular conduction. Exaggeration of these effects can occur particularly in patients with impaired ventricular function and/or SA or AV conduction abnormalities. Neither medicine should therefore be administered intravenously within 48 hours of discontinuing the other.

Nebivolol and Anti-arrhythmics

Caution should be exercised when administering beta-blockers with Class I anti-arrhythmic drugs and amiodarone as their effect on atrial conduction time and their negative inotropic effect may be potentiated. Such interactions can have life threatening consequences.

Nebivolol and Clonidine

Beta-blockers increase the risk of rebound hypertension after sudden withdrawal of chronic clonidine treatment.

Nebivolol and Digoxin

Digitalis glycosides associated with beta-blockers may increase atrio-ventricular conduction times. Nebivolol does not influence the kinetics of digoxin and clinical trials have not shown any evidence of an interaction.

Nebivolol and Oral Antidiabetic Drugs

Glucose levels are unaffected, however symptoms of hypoglycaemia may be masked.

HIGHLIGHTS

Nebivolol can be safely co-administred with most of the drugs used for the treatment of patients with metabolic syndrome. However, potential interactions can occur when nebivolol is co-administred with calcium channel antagonists. Caution should be exercised when nebivol, like all the beta-blockers, is prescribed together with oral Hypoglycemc agents, since symptoms of hypoglycaemia may be masked.

ALPHA-BLOCKERS

Doxazosin

Brief Compound Description

Doxazosin mesylate 1-(4-amino-6,7-dimethoxy-2-quinazolinyl)-4- (1,4-benzodioxan-2-ylcarbonyl) piperazine methanesulfonate. The structural formula is:

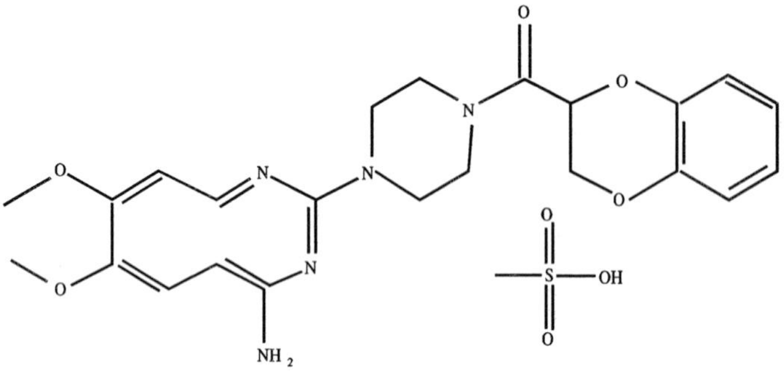

O
N
O
O
N
N
O
S OH
N
O
O
O
NH 2

Drug Interactions

Doxazosin and Thiazide Diuretics, Beta-blocking Agents, and NSAIDs Drugs

Doxazosin mesylate has been administered without any evidence of an adverse drug interaction to patients receiving thiazide diuretics, beta-blocking agents, and NSAIDs drugs.

Doxazosin and Phosphodiesterase 5 Inhibitors

Tadalafil augmented the hypotensive effects of doxazosin but had little hemodynamic interaction with tamsulosin.

Doxazosin and Digoxin, Warfarin, or Indomethacin

Most (98%) of plasma doxazosin is protein bound. *In vitro* data in human plasma indicate that doxazosin mesylate has no effect on protein binding of digoxin, warfarin, or indomethacin.

ALPHA (2)-ADRENOCEPTOR AGONISTS

Clonidine

Brief Compound Description

Clonidine hydrochloride USP) is a centrally acting alpha-agonist hypotensive agent. Clonidine hydrochloride is an imidazoline derivative and exists as a mesomeric compound. The chemical name is 2-(2,6-dichlorophenylamino)-2-imidazoline hydrochloride. The following is the structural formula

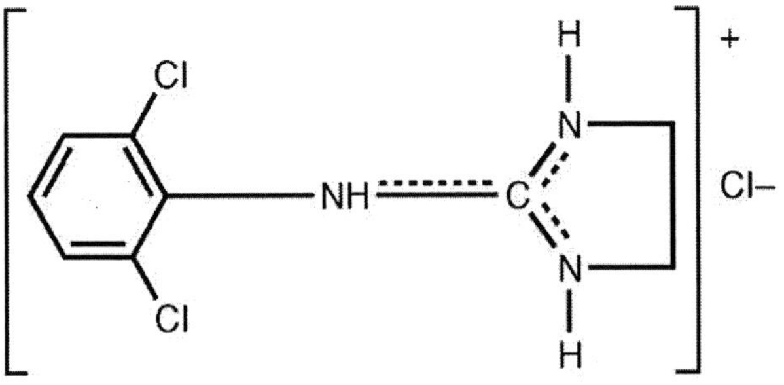

$C_9H_9Cl_2N_3 \cdot HCl$ Mol. Wt. 266.56

Mechanism of Action

Clonidine stimulates alpha-adrenoreceptors in the brain stem. This action results in reduced sympathetic outflow from the central nervous system and in decreases in peripheral resistance, renal vascular resistance, heart rate, and blood pressure.

Drug Interactions

Clonidine and Digoxin, Calcium Channel Blockers and Beta-blockers

Due to a potential for additive effects such as bradycardia and AV block, caution is warranted in patients receiving clonidine concomitantly with agents known to affect sinus node function or AV nodal conduction, e.g. digitalis, calcium channel blockers and beta-blockers.

Clonidine and Oral Hypoglycaemic Agents

Clonidine induced a dose-dependent hyperglycemic response in fed rats. The hyperglycemic response induced by clonidine and other alpha-2 adrenergic agonists is mediated by alpha-2 adrenergic receptors located within the central nervous system and clonidine-induced hyperglycemia is affected by enhanced gluconeogenesis [1].

References

[1] DiTullio NW, Cieslinski L, Matthews WD, Storer B Mechanisms involved in the hyperglycemic response induced by clonidine and other alpha-2 adrenoceptor agonists. *J Pharmacol Exp Ther.* 1984Jan;228(1):168-73.

CENTRAL IMIDAZOLINE (I1)-RECEPTORS AGONIST

Moxonidine

The structural formula of moxonidine is the following:

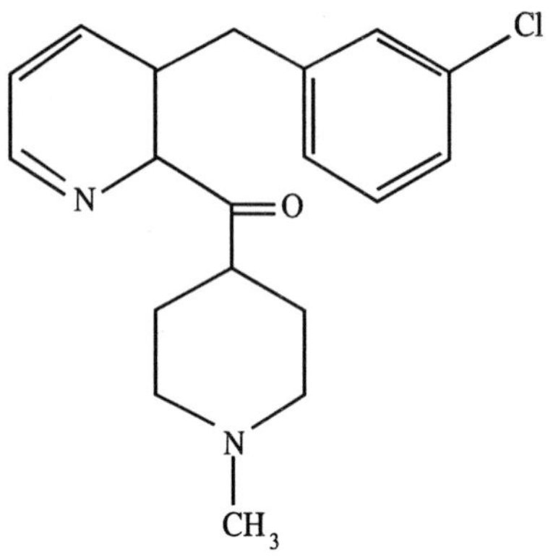

Mechanism of Action

Moxonidine is a second generation centrally-acting antihypertensive which act as an agonist of the imidazoline I1 receptor in brainstem sympathetic nuclei. Moxonidine is a centrally active imidazoline receptor agonist that effectively lowers blood pressure and has been shown to have beneficial effects on lipid and carbohydrate metabolism. Moxonidin is the effective antyhypertensive drug positively effecting on metabolism in patients with obesity [1]. It is thought to stimulate imidazoline receptors in the brain. When moxonidine acts on these receptors it causes the blood vessels to relax and widen. Moxonidine is also thought to have an effect on other receptors called alpha-2 receptors. These receptors are found in the brain. By binding to these receptors moxonidine prevents the release of other chemicals in the brain that would normally act to increase blood pressure.

Drug Interactions

Monoxidine and Inhibitory Cannabinoid CB1 Receptors

The cross-antagonism of imidazoline receptor agonists/antagonists with CB1 receptor antagonists/agonists suggests that these receptors may have certain binding domains in common or that they interact with each other in an unknown manner [2].

Monoxidine and Hydrochlorothiazide

No interactions occurred when moxonidine 0.4 mg o.d. has been administred in combination with hydrochlorothiazide [3].

Monoxidine and Glibenclamide

No substantial pharmacokinetic interactions between these drugs have been described. Regarding the influence of glibenclamide on the pharmacokinetics of moxonidine, no significant changes were seen. In the presence of moxonidine, a minor decrease of bioavailability of glibenclamide was detectable but the differences were small and not considered to be of clinical significance [4].

Monoxidine and Quinidine

Quinidine does not affect the renal clearance of moxonidine. The decrease in apparent total clearance of moxonidine with quinidine coadministration was possibly due to metabolic inhibition, though not likely to be clinically significant [5].

References

[1] Sharma AM, Wagner T, Marsalek P. Moxonidine in the treatment of overweight and obese patients with the metabolic syndrome: a postmarketing surveillance study. *J Hum Hypertens. 2004* Sep;18(9):669-75

[2] Molderings GJ, Likungu J, Gothert M Presynaptic cannabinoid and imidazoline receptors in the human heart and their potential relationship. *Naunyn Schmiedebergs Arch Pharmacol.* 1999 Aug;360(2):157-64.

[3] Frei M, Kuster L, Gardosch von Krosigk PP, Koch HF, Kuppers H. Moxonidine and hydrochlorothiazide in combination: a synergistic antihypertensive effect. *J Cardiovasc Pharmacol.* 1994;24 Suppl 1:S25-8.

[4] Muller M, Weimann HJ, Eden G, Weber W, Michaelis K, Dilger C, Achtert G. Steady state investigation of possible pharmacokinetic interactions of moxonidine and glibenclamide. *Eur J Drug Metab Pharmacokinet.* 1993 Jul-Sep;18(3):277-83.

[5] Wise SD, Chan C, Schaefer HG, He MM, Pouliquen IJ, Mitchell MI. Quinidine does not affect the renal clearance of moxonidine. *Br J Clin Pharmacol.* 2002 Sep;54(3):251-4.

DIURETICS

Furosemide

Brief Compound Description

Furosemide is a diuretic which is an anthranilic acid derivative. Chemically, it is 4-chloro- N -furfuryl-5-sulfamoylanthranilic acid. The structural formula is:

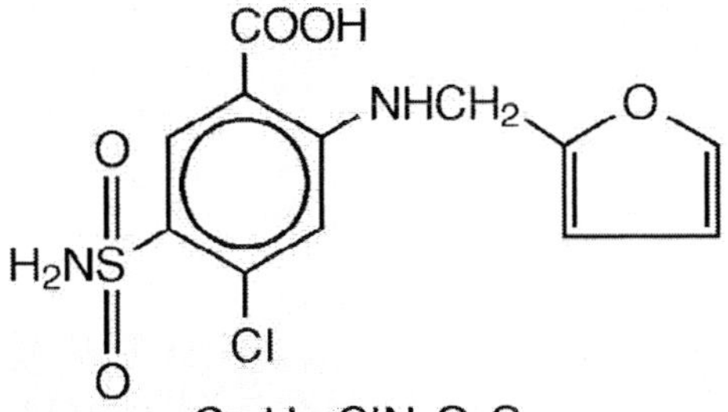

$C_{12}H_{11}ClN_2O_5S$

M.W. 330.75

Mechanism of Action

Furosemide inhibits primarily the reabsorption of sodium and chloride not only in the proximal and distal tubules but also in the loop of Henle. The high degree of efficacy is largely due to this unique site of action. The action on the distal tubule is independent of any inhibitory effect on carbonic anhydrase and aldosterone. Recent evidence suggests that furosemide glucuronide is the only or at least the major biotransformation product of furosemide in man. Furosemide is extensively bound to plasma proteins, mainly to albumin. The onset of diuresis following oral administration is within one hour. The peak effect occurs within the first or second hour. The duration of diuretic effect is 6 to 8 hours

Drug Interactions

Furosemide and antihypertensive drugs Furosemide may add to or potentiate the therapeutic effect of other antihypertensive drugs. Furosemide may decrease arterial responsiveness to norepinephrine. However, norepinephrine may still be used effectively.

Furosemide and sucralfate Simultaneous administration of sucralfate and furosemide tablets may reduce the natriuretic and antihypertensive effects of furosemide. Patients receiving both drugs should be observed closely to determine if the desired diuretic and/or antihypertensive effect of furosemide is achieved. The intake of furosemide and sucralfate should be separated by at least two hours.

Furosemide and NSAIDs Combination of furosemide and acetylsalicylic acid temporarily reduced creatinine clearance in patients with chronic renal insufficiency. Coadministration of indomethacin may reduce the natriuretic and antihypertensive effects of furosemide in some patients by inhibiting prostaglandin synthesis. Indomethacin may also affect plasma renin levels, aldosterone excretion and renin profile evaluation. Patients receiving both indomethacin and furosemide should be observed closely to determine if the desired diuretic and/or antihypertensive effect of furosemide is achieved.

Hydrochlorothiazide

Brief Compound Description

Hydrochlorothiazide has the empirical formula $C_7H_8ClN_3O_4S_2$ and a molecular weight of 297.75. It is chemically described as 2 H -1,2,4-Benzothiadiazine-7-sulfonamide,6-chloro-3,4-dihydro-,1,1-dioxide. Hydrochlorothiazide is a thiazide diuretic and its structural formula is:

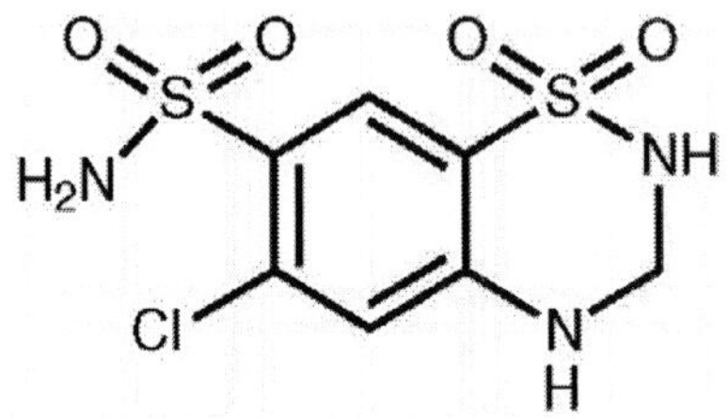

Mechanism of Action

The mechanism of the antihypertensive effect of thiazides is unknown. Thiazides do not usually affect normal blood pressure. Hydrochlorothiazide is a diuretic and antihypertensive. It affects the distal renal tubular mechanism of electrolyte reabsorption. Hydrochlorothiazide increases excretion of sodium and chloride in approximately equivalent amounts. Natriuresis may be accompanied by some loss of potassium and bicarbonate.

Drug Interactions

Table 1. Potential drug-drug interactions with hydrochlorothiazide in metabolic syndrome

YES	Mechanism and effect	NO
Oral hypoglycemic agents	increased glucose	Ace-inhibitors Sartans
Cholestyramine	⇓reduced absorption of hydrochlorothiazide	

Hydrochlorothiazide and Antidiabetic Drugs

In case of coadministration of Hydrochlorothiazide with Antidiabetic drugs dosage adjustment of the antidiabetic drug may be required. Hydrochlorothiazide significantly increased fasting glucose and glycosylated haemoglobin (HbA1c) [1].

Hydrochlorothiazide and ACE-inhibitors

Fosinopril and Hydrochlorothiazide in a combination display pharmacokinetic profiles similar to those achieved when either drug is administered alone or when coadministered in separate tablets. When used with Hydrochlorothiazide, the favorable pharmacokinetic feature of fosinopril, dual and compensatory pathways of renal and hepatic elimination, is preserved [2].

Hydrochlorothiazide and Cholestyramine and Colestipol Resins

Absorption of hydrochlorothiazide is impaired in the presence of anionic exchange resins. Single doses of either cholestyramine or colestipol resins bind the hydrochlorothiazide and reduce its absorption from the gastrointestinal tract by up to 85 and 43 percent, respectively.

References

[1] Dornhorst A, Powell SH, Pensky J. Aggravation by propranolol of hyperglycaemic effect of hydrochlorothiazide in type II diabetics without alteration of insulin secretion. *Lancet.* 1985 Jan 19;1(8421):123-6.

[2] Uderman HD, Much DR, Brennan J, Delaney CL, Morgenthien EA, Weaver J, Stouffer BC, Chang SY, VanHarken D, Liao W Fosinopril and hydrochlorothiazide combination versus individual components: lack of a pharmacokinetic interaction. *Ann Pharmacother. 1999* May;33(5):525-30.

POTASSIUM-SPARING DIURETICS

Amiloride

Brief Compound Description

Amiloride HCl, an antikaliuretic-diuretic agent, is a pyrazine-carbonyl-guanidine that is unrelated chemically to other known antikaliuretic or diuretic agents. It is designated chemically as 3,5-diamino-6-chloro- N -(diaminomethylene) pyrazinecarboxamide monohydrochloride, dihydrate and has a molecular weight of 302.12. Its empirical formula is $C_6H_8ClN_7O \cdot HCl \cdot 2H_2O$ and its structural formula is:

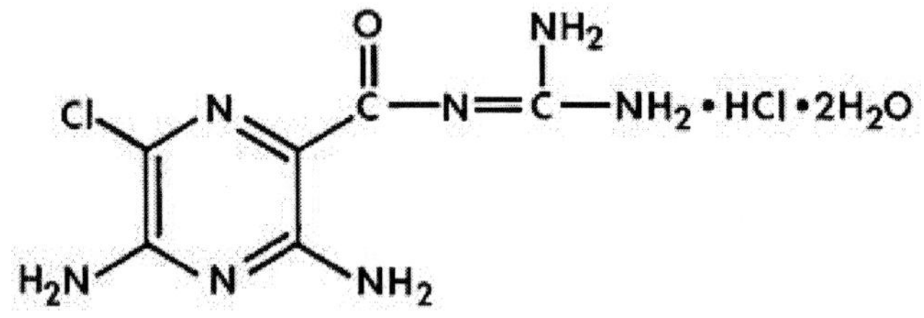

Mechanism of Action

Amilorideis a potassium-conserving (antikaliuretic) drug that possesses weak (compared with thiazide diuretics) natriuretic, diuretic, and antihypertensive activity. These effects have been partially additive to the effects of thiazide diuretics in some clinical studies. When administered with a thiazide or loop diuretic, Amiloride has been shown to decrease the enhanced urinary excretion of magnesium which occurs when a thiazide or loop diuretic is used alone. Amiloride has potassium-conserving activity in patients receiving kaliuretic-diuretic agents. Amiloride is not an aldosterone antagonist and its effects are seen even in the absence of aldosterone. Amiloride exerts its potassium sparing effect through the inhibition of sodium reabsorption at the distal convoluted tubule, cortical collecting tubule and collecting duct; this decreases the net negative potential of the tubular lumen and reduces both potassium and hydrogen secretion and their subsequent excretion. This mechanism accounts in large part for the potassium sparing action of amiloride.

Drug Interactions

Amiloride and ACE Inhibitors

When amiloride HCl is administered concomitantly with an angiotensin-converting enzyme inhibitor, an angiotensin II receptor antagonist, the risk of hyperkalemia may be increased. Therefore, if concomitant use of these agents is indicated because of demonstrated hypokalemia, they should be used with caution and with frequent monitoring of serum potassium

Amiloride and NSAIDs

In some patients, the administration of a non-steroidal anti-inflammatory agent can reduce the diuretic, natriuretic, and antihypertensive effects of loop, potassium-sparing and thiazide diuretics. Therefore, when amiloride and non-steroidal anti-inflammatory agents are used concomitantly, the patient should be observed closely to determine if the desired effect of the diuretic is obtained.

Triamterene

Brief Compound Description

Triamterene is 2, 4, 7-triamino-6-phenyl-pteridine. Its molecular weight is 253.27. The structural formula is:

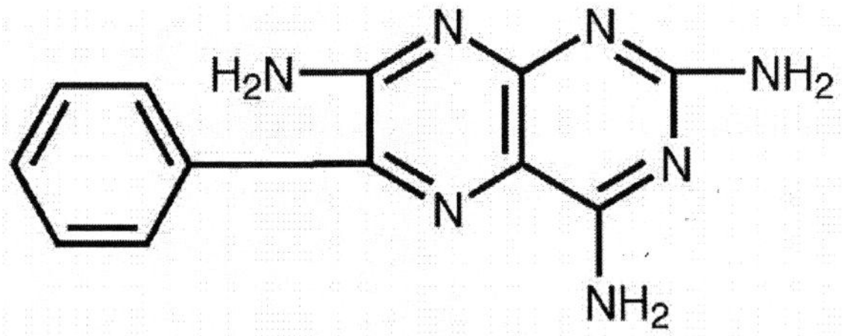

Triamterene

Mechanism of Action

Triamterene has a unique mode of action; it inhibits the reabsorption of sodium ions in exchange for potassium and hydrogen ions at that segment of the distal tubule under the control of adrenal mineralocorticoids (especially aldosterone). This activity is not directly related to aldosterone secretion or antagonism; it is a result of a direct effect on the renal tubule.

Drug Interactions

Triamterene and ACE Inhibitors

Potassium-sparing agents should be used with caution in conjunction with angiotensin-converting enzyme (ACE) inhibitors due to an increased risk of hyperkalemia

Triamterene and NSAIDs

A possible interaction resulting in acute renal failure has been reported in a few subjects when indomethacin, a nonsteroidal anti-inflammatory agent, was given with triamterene. Caution is advised in administering nonsteroidal anti-inflammatory agents with triamterene.

Triamterene and Antidiabetes Drugs

Triamterene may raise blood glucose levels; for adult onset diabetes, dosage adjustments of hypoglycemic agents may be necessary during and after therapy; concurrent use with chlorpropamide may increase the risk of severe hyponatremia.

Spironolactone

Brief Compound Description

Spironolactone, 17-hydroxy-7alpha-mercapto-3-oxo-17alpha-pregn-4-ene-21-carboxylic acid gamma lactone acetate, which has the following structural formula:

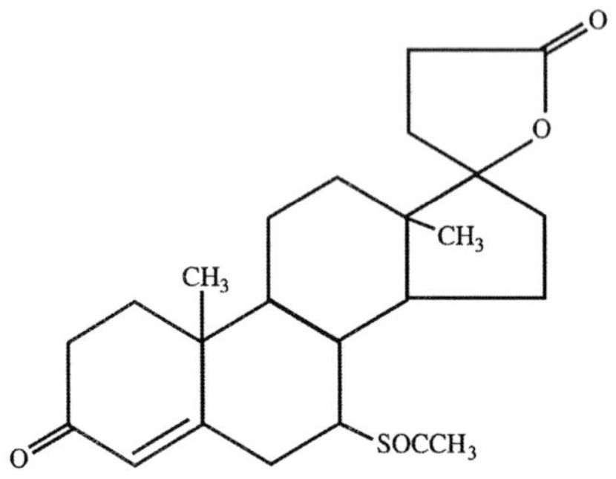

Mechanism of Action

Spironolactone is a specific pharmacologic antagonist of aldosterone, acting primarily through competitive binding of receptors at the aldosterone-dependent sodium-potassium exchange site in the distal convoluted renal tubule. Spironolactone scauses increased amounts of sodium and water to be excreted, while potassium is retained. Spironolactone acts both as a diuretic and as an antihypertensive drug by this mechanism. It may be given alone or with other diuretic agents which act more proximally in the renal tubule.

Drug Interactions

Spironolactone and ACE Inhibitors

Concomitant administration of ACE inhibitors with potassium-sparing diuretics has been associated with severe hyperkalemia.

Sprinolactone and NSAIDs

Nonsteroidal anti-inflammatory drugs (NSAIDs): In some patients, the administration of an NAISD can reduce the diuretic, natriuretic, and antihypertensive effect of loop, potassium-sparing and thiazide diuretics. Combination of NSAIDs, eg, indomethacin, with potassium-sparing diuretics has been associated with severe hyperkalemia.

Spironolactone and Digoxin

Spironolactone has been shown to increase the half life of digoxin. This may result in increased serum.

INDEX

A

B

C

D

N

O

P

Q

R